# La Doctora

## The Journal of an American Doctor
## Practicing Medicine on the Amazon River

# La Doctora

*The Journal of an American Doctor*
*Practicing Medicine on the Amazon River*

**Linnea Smith, M.D.**

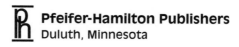

**Pfeifer-Hamilton Publishers**
Duluth, Minnesota

Pfeifer-Hamilton Publishers
210 West Michigan
Duluth, MN 55802-1908
218-727-0500
E-mail: books1@phpublisher.com
Web site: http://www.phpublisher.com

*La Doctora: The Journal of an American Doctor*
*Practicing Medicine on the Amazon River*

Printed in Canada
by Friesens
Altona, Manitoba

10   9   8   7   6   5   4   3   2   1

Associate Editor: Casey McGee
Art Director: Joy Morgan Dey

Library of Congress Cataloging-in-Publication Data
Smith, Linnea
        La doctora: the journal of an American doctor
        practicing medicine on the Amazon River/Linnea
        Smith
        240 p.   20.5 cm.
    ISBN 1-57025-140-1 (pbk.)
    1. Smith, Linnea.  2. Physicians--Amazon River Region--
Biography.  3. Tropical medicine--Amazon River Region--
Anecdotes.  4. Indians of South America--Amazon River
Region--Medical care--Anecdotes.  I. Title.
        R483.S55 A3 1999
        610'.92--ddc21
        [B]
                                                        98-40076
                                                          CIP

# Dedication

To Pam, without whose friendship I never would have made it through my first year here, and who upon reading my journal came running down the path waving the volume over her head and shouting, "You've got a book here!"

To Dan and Judy, who probably got more than they bargained for when they walked into my houseplant store many years ago, and without whose assistance and management of my life in general I would not be able to continue staying here.

# Acknowledgments

It is impossible to thank all those who have helped me with this book, let alone the many who have made it possible for me to live and work where I do. I therefore ask forgiveness for any omissions.

Thanks must go first and foremost to Dan and Judy Peterson, who not only manage the Amazon Medical Project, but also take care of the remnants of my life in Wisconsin—including, but not by any means limited to, a major renovation of my house during my absence. Equally first on the list should be Peter Jenson and his Explorama Tours, who have provided my food, shelter, social life, transport, and moral support in Peru for the last eight years. Their guests also provide much of the funding for the ongoing operations of the clinic, as well as the contact with my former world that keeps me from feeling completely isolated. Pam Bucur of Explorama also merits top billing for being my friend, to say the least.

Support for the clinic comes from so many different people that it is impossible to thank them all, but Paul Gakle's efforts in writing grant proposals have kept the clinic financially viable for the past few years. Many individuals and groups have made contributions of funds and/or medicines. Jon Helstrom spearheaded efforts by the Duluth, Minnesota, and Thunder Bay, Ontario, Canada, Rotary Clubs and, in turn, inspired other clubs to move me from a single room in a house with a thatched roof out to the "real clinic" on the riverbank. As District 5580, they provided the clinic facility; as individuals, they have given friendship and other support that has gone far beyond their building program.

My parents deserve, and receive, my deepest thanks and appreciation. They not only put up with raising me and then seeing me run off to the jungle, but they also continue to help with the

Amazon Medical Project and with my personal needs, such as providing a home to return to. My sister Betsy and her husband Brian also have devoted countless hours to keeping up with a growing stack of correspondence.

Finally, thanks must go to Pfeifer-Hamilton Publishers, specifically Don Tubesing and Casey McGee. They not only signed up a nonauthor to write this book, they also gave me unlimited latitude in what I wanted to say and how I wanted to say it. I didn't know that publishers did that, but they have.

For those of you who feel inclined to help support the clinic, the Amazon Medical Project is a tax-exempt, nonprofit organization. Donations to it are tax-deductible, and since Dan and Judy Peterson and my family do most of the managing, virtually all contributions go directly to maintaining the clinic. The address is:

**Amazon Medical Project**
**5372 Mahocker Road, Mazomanie, Wisconsin 53560**
**Fax 608-795-2646**
**e-mail address: amp@amazonmedical.org**
**Website: www.amazonmedical.org**

Any of you who are inspired to visit us here may contact Explorama by e-mail at <amazon@explorama.com> or visit their website at www.explorama.com.

# Table of Contents

**More Jungle Medicine**

**The End of the Beginning**

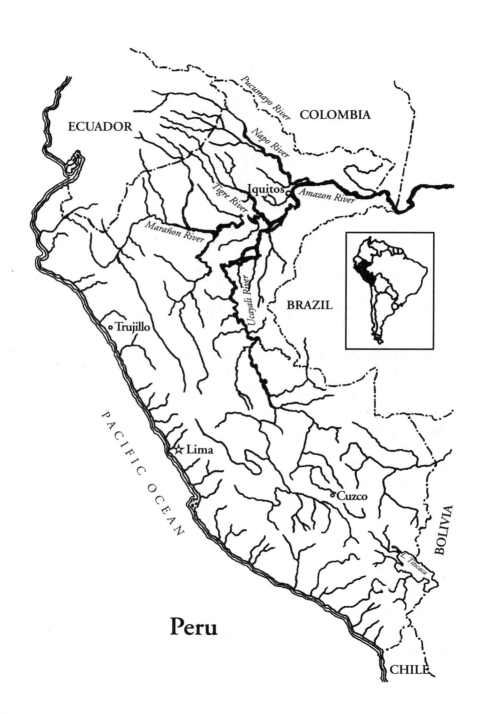

CHAPTER ONE

# "My Wife
# Can't Have Her Baby!"

**The Amazon River jungle—Yanamono, Peru**

"My wife can't have her baby. You must come!"

The young man standing at the stream's edge had simple fear in his eyes and a desperate plea in his voice. It was early in the morning and the clinic was not yet officially open, but babies trying to be born do not always respect clinic hours. The mere fact that he and the elderly midwife accompanying him had paddled their dugout canoe from the far side of the island to the small stream where my rudimentary clinic was located indicated that there was a problem.

And this one would turn out to be significant.

It always makes me nervous when people show up on my doorstep, wanting me to make a housecall. No matter how they describe the problem they want me to attend, it is never the way the patient actually looks when I arrive, so I never know what to expect once I reach the humble abode I am being summoned to. Obstetrical housecalls make me even more nervous.

So I was immediately and especially nervous that morning when a dugout canoe pulled up bearing a young man and an old woman, both with furrowed brows, who wanted me to go with them to their home on Yanamono Island because "My wife can't have her baby."

On television, babies are born in the back of taxicabs with no more than a few mild hysterics; in real life, usually things work out fairly smoothly. Women, after all, have been having babies since long before doctors were invented. However, obstetrical problems, when they do occur, can escalate rapidly into life-and-death situations. Hemorrhage, pain, seizures, death—all sorts of truly unpleasant things—can happen unexpectedly and very messily to a young and otherwise healthy woman. It is one thing to deal with complications of childbirth in a modern hospital with nurses, anesthesiologists, and other doctors ready to assist at a moment's notice, and with facilities such as operating rooms, running water, electric lighting, and blood transfusion services. But out here alone, in the jungle, with none of those support technologies or services, any complication could mean trouble.

Women around here generally have their babies at home under the supervision and assistance of a midwife, often their mother or mother-in-law, and everything normally goes quite smoothly. When a midwife throws in the towel it's usually because of a real problem with the delivery. Clearly, in this case, the midwife didn't think she could help.

My only formal obstetric training lasted six weeks, as part of my third year in medical school. Anticipating the need for some rudimentary childbirth skills, before I left home I had collared a surgeon friend for some hasty instructions on surgical procedures for emergencies. "Oh, it's easy, Linnea, you can do it," he said blithely. He outlined the pertinent anatomy, mentioned one or two pitfalls to watch for, and had me observe him from ten feet away as he performed a couple of cesarean sections. And that was the total extent of my OB-Gyn training—not a lot, if I were to be faced with a real emergency. This went through my head in the seconds following the would-be father's announcement.

I had always known that some day, far from any backup, it would be a matter of do or die—me doing or the patient dying. But how could I take on that responsibility when I felt so thoroughly unprepared? So those words, "My wife can't have her baby," struck fear into my heart. I didn't think I was ready.

Ready or not, however, here I went.

The young man and his wife, Isabel, lived on the far side of Yanamono Island: two hours away paddling the dugout, or forty-five minutes by motorboat—which was generously offered by one of Explorama's guides. I quickly packed the supplies that I thought I would need, posted a note on the clinic door saying that I was away on an emergency, and joined the would-be father and the elderly midwife on their journey back across the Amazon River to the other side of the island.

When we arrived, three and a half hours after her husband had left to summon me, Isabel was having normal contractions again. As far as I could tell, everything seemed to be OK.

"OK" in obstetric terms means she was having strong contractions at a regular rate, her blood pressure was normal, there was no hemorrhaging, the baby was head down, and I could hear its heart beating. The cervix, or opening to the uterus, wasn't dilated as far as it would need to be, but it was beginning to open, and the amniotic sac was still unbroken. Isabel looked tired but otherwise fine. I tried to reassure the family with these findings, but they were worried. A neighbor of theirs had died a few nights earlier, giving birth to twins, and they thought that Isabel's labor looked similar. Nevertheless, I really couldn't suggest anything to do right now but wait. So I encouraged them to let me know if any problems arose or if her contractions stopped once again, and I prepared to return to the clinic.

I was making motions to leave when I noticed with some surprise that the family, too, were packing their belongings. Obviously, they had decided to bring Isabel back with me. Well, practically speaking, it would be difficult for me to return here later or for them to call me—what could they have done, picked up a telephone in their palm-slat hut and called 911? And if she did have more trouble, her chances would probably be better at the clinic.

However, what I optimistically called "the clinic" was at that time one small room, about eight by twelve feet, in one of Explorama's thatch-roofed houses. Lighting was courtesy of kerosene lantern, bats roosted underneath the table that I used for a desk, and running water was what happened when I filled a pitcher at the stream or at one of Explorama's showers and tipped it. I had virtually no instruments, and not even an exam table, only a single bed with a cloth-covered pad. Furthermore, Explorama Lodge, although kind enough to let me locate my services there, is first and foremost a tourist destination and was at that moment hosting the first-ever International Rainforest Conference, with over 170 attendees in a facility built to accommodate about 120 people. How would they feel about a woman in labor during their workshops focused on studying birds and fish? Worse, how would they feel if the woman died right in their midst? It really didn't seem like a good idea to bring her along.

However, the family had already made the decision, with or without my concurrence. We all filed down to the boat, settled Isabel on the floor, and journeyed back to my clinic at Explorama Lodge.

Three hours later, we were still awaiting the baby's arrival. It was my great good fortune that one of the lodge's guests was a family practice doctor, Ward Powers. He said he hadn't done OB for years, but when I sought him out to get a second opinion on the progress of Isabel's labor, he readily came along. He examined her and agreed that since she seemed OK, it was best to just wait. Sounded good to me, especially as there wasn't much else we could have done.

Darkness came, and still no baby. The contractions were strong and continued at nice normal two-minute intervals, and at four in the afternoon, her water finally broke with a rush. At that point I thought, aha!—now we'll have a baby. But the head still didn't seem to be descending. Normally, with each contraction, the fetus comes a little farther down, until finally the baby pops out altogether. The progress may be very slow (and usually seems interminable to the woman in labor), but over time the movement downward should be noticeable.

Workshop participants were meeting in the open area just outside the clinic, and I was grateful and relieved that Isabel was tremendously stoic. Not a murmur from her the whole time, even though she was convinced she would die, just as her neighbor had done. She even made a few jokes in the intervals between her pains. But I was getting really worried, and didn't want to wait until the middle of the night to find out that there was going to be a catastrophe.

My little "clinic," although comfortably familiar to me, was drastically underprepared for a surgical procedure, particularly at night without the benefit of electric lights. The warm glow of kerosene lamps may be cozy and romantic, but they aren't very effective as surgical operating lights, and I couldn't imagine doing any complex surgical procedure by flashlight—especially not a complex surgical procedure that I had never performed before. It was time to get out of there and start the one-and-a-half-hour journey to the nearest medical center, twenty-five miles upriver at the town of Indiana. There was no doctor there—I had been fulfilling that role on a sporadic basis—but the people who worked there knew me, and there was an operating table, and surgical instruments, and with a little luck, probably even electric light—if we could get there, that was.

Getting somewhere rapidly in the jungle is easier said than done, especially at night. There are no cars here, no roads, no MedFlight. We had no radio, either, but whom could we have called anyway?—ambulance service by river? The solution eventually came from Explorama: the lodge was so full with the workshop that the press contingent was staying upriver just beyond Indiana. They generously granted us permission to ride along in the boat that would take them on the trip upriver.

The medical center at Indiana had decent instruments, but I knew from working there that anything disposable would not likely be in very good shape. I grabbed a bag of IV fluid, some suture material, scalpel blades, and a few pairs of surgical gloves, and we boarded the banana boat, now our emergency water-taxi. Ward Powers came by to see how things were going, and offered to join us. I could have hugged him; I had been hoping his interest would be piqued, because I really needed the moral support, but had been reluctant to ask him to go along on what might well prove to be a nightmare. As it turned out, the medical procedure that would follow would have been impossible without him.

I felt at least a little bit better for having reached a decision. At Indiana there would be more light, more hands, more room, more instruments, and fewer tourists. And if my patient still wasn't a mom by the time we arrived, I would feel assured that something was drastically wrong and that a surgical delivery would be in order. I felt a bit like Butterfly McQueen's character in *Gone with the Wind*; "Oh sure, I can do a cesarean, no problem. No problem a-tall."

The riverboat ride quickly turned into a bad dream. Isabel lay in back on the wooden bench, moaning quietly, still with contractions every two minutes. The night was stormy, and the river was full of floating debris and worse—once when we hit something, the motor stopped. While Gato, the spare boat driver, went back to the motor and sorted it out, Luís, the *motorista* (driver), crawled out on the bow and pushed us away from the huge floating tree with which we had somehow become entangled and which was pushing us back downriver.

The press people with whom we were hitchhiking did their best to restrain their instincts to crowd in on our patient with their lights and cameras. Still, they were press, and they wanted to document the story. They kept saying, now, we don't want to be intrusive or anything, at the same time that they were standing on tiptoe and shining their klieg lights on the moaning Isabel. We distracted them for a while with interviews with Ward and me, but I finally had to ask them to turn off all their gear and get out of the way, since Luís could hardly see where he was going because of the reflected light from behind him. There are no headlights on the boats, no street lamps on the river, and with the rain, the spotlight Luís was using didn't reach more than fifty feet. It's dangerous enough on this river at night without being blinded by the glare of television camera lights.

The clinic at Indiana is staffed by *auxiliares*, equivalent to LPNs in their training and often extremely capable, in the years when they have no doctor they have to do everything—examine, diagnose, prescribe medicines, sew up lacerations, and—of course— deliver babies. When we finally arrived at Indiana, I raced up the walk. I flew past Nirma, the *auxiliare* on duty that night, headed straight for the surgery room, and flipped the switch to turn on the single ceiling light. Nothing. I turned to Nirma. "Burned out," she noted, shrugging and smiling in her usual cheerful, passive, thoroughly unmotivated way. I cursed in English. Nirma is a nice person, but not someone with much sense of urgency or initiative. Besides, there probably wasn't a spare lightbulb around anyway, nor was there a ladder to get up and change it if we did have a new bulb. In this room there is one tall narrow window, but that doesn't supply much light at night.

By this time the others had carried our patient up the riverbank and into the clinic. Her delivery still had not progressed—that is, the baby's head was no farther down than it had been before we left—and the situation was now becoming desperate. Mothers-to-be often sleep between contractions, but Isabel wasn't sleeping, she was losing consciousness between contractions and becoming more and more delirious even while awake. She didn't have much time left.

We helped her onto the surgery table, and I turned to Ward. "What do you think? Where do we work—Here in darkness, by kerosene lamp, or in the office where there's a light but no operating table?" He thought for a moment, then wisely pointed out that the table was probably movable. It was. We dragged it, with our patient still on it, around the corner to the office/exam room, where a single fluorescent lamp beamed as well as it could, in the center of the ten- or twelve-foot-high ceiling.

For anesthesia, we had only lidocaine and ketamine. Lidocaine is a local anesthetic (and the surgeon who had assured me I could easily do a cesarean had also casually tossed out the observation that "you could do it just with local, if you had to"). Ketamine is a general anesthetic, which means it puts you to sleep.

The problems with general anesthesia are several. Mostly, these are drugs that have a narrow therapeutic to toxic ratio— the amount needed to knock you out temporarily is perilously close to the amount that would knock you out permanently. This problem, in a modern medical facility, is surmounted by carefully monitoring the patient with complex equipment, managed by a well-trained anesthesiologist, and by using a combination of drugs, including some to put the patient to sleep, others to block pain, and still others to paralyze— the latter group, by the way, derived from the poisons on the hunting darts used by Indians in this area of the Amazon.

Enter ketamine. Developed in the 1960s, it quickly caught on as a general anesthetic that does not (USUALLY does not) stop the patient from breathing. This means that an anesthesiologist and a whole bunch of machinery and monitoring equipment are not needed, an ideal situation for low-tech applications. Ketamine fell out of favor in the U.S. when it was found to be quite similar to the horse tranquilizer phencyclidine, sold on the street as "angel dust," and to cause horrendous hallucinations and vivid dreams as the patient awakens. It remains useful, however, for children, who seem less susceptible to the hallucinatory awakenings, and in countries where the alternatives are few or none.

Such as this particular country, at this particular moment. Given the choice between wild hallucinations, or death due to the baby who couldn't get out of her belly, I didn't care if Isabel had funny dreams.

There was a partially filled vial of ketamine at the medical center—an inadequate dose, but by now, with all the time that had elapsed and all the travel and jostling around she had been through, Isabel was already so close to death that we probably could have operated on her with only lidocaine, or maybe even with nothing.

So I injected what little ketamine we had on hand into her right antecubital vein and taped the syringe in place, took a deep breath, and pulled on sterile gloves. The left one promptly tore across the palm. I glared at it and snapped at Nirma to bring another. She handed me the last one there was. Ward was already gloved. It never occurred to either one of us to scrub our hands as we would normally do before surgery, nor to put on masks and gowns, since there were none. We used the office desk as the table on which we set out the instruments.

Then we began.

I picked up the scalpel. Ward stabilized the skin. I cut. The subcutaneous fat welled up, and I sliced through that. It took a while to pick up and cut through the preperitoneal fat, which sits just in front of the cobweb-thin peritoneal membrane. Inside the peritoneal membrane lie the intestines, with the other digestive organs above and our goal—the uterus—below. I kept thinking the fat was peritoneum, but it was too thick, and Ward kept saying no, I don't think we're through yet, till finally the micro-thin peritoneum was under the scissors tips, and then we located the swollen uterus. To my immense relief, it suddenly bulged out where a miniature foot kicked in protest. The baby was still alive!

I don't remember exactly when we started sweating in earnest, but I do remember sweat dripping off my elbows, and I recall Ward asking for help to defog his glasses.

The bladder pushed itself up. I remembered my surgeon friend saying to push it down off the uterus and cut a little above it. That move allows the bladder to roll back over the incision and seal off the scar from the intestines. But it seemed easier (and the uterine location seemed right) just to cut a centimeter or two above the bladder and parallel to it. I did remember to stay away from the uterine arteries, running along each side of the uterus—cut one of those, and your patient may hemorrhage to death, if you can't find it and close it off in time. I carefully avoided them as well as the ureters, those tiny but essential tubes that run from the kidneys to the bladder. The incision seemed too small for our work, and I cautiously extended it.

Suddenly, amidst all the blood, there was the baby, smooth shoulders visible through the incision in the uterus.

I reached down to find the head and felt the wetted-down fur of baby hair. But I couldn't get my hand around it, and couldn't budge it. I withdrew, and appealed to Ward. He tried . . . no success, either. The baby's head was by now too firmly lodged in the mother's pelvis.

Once I realized that, I said to hell with sterile technique. Such a decision is medical heresy. In training we were constantly reminded that it does no good to complete an operation only to have the patient die a few days later of infection introduced by the surgeon. On the other hand, it does no good at all, I reasoned, to abide by the sacredness of sterile techniques and watch both the baby and the mother die on the spot. It was by now absolutely clear that this baby was not at any time going to pass through his mother's pelvis. There were two and only two options: either the baby would exit through her abdomen—or they would both die soon. This comforting thought enabled me to temporarily regard sterile technique as a disposable nicety that neither of our two patients could at the moment afford.

I reached down with my right hand into the vagina and gave a firm push upward on the baby's head…and pop! He was finally free. I reached back into the abdominal incision, slid the fingers of my left hand now easily around the head, and pulled backward and up, and after all this trauma, suddenly there was a baby in my hands.

He looked fairly blue to me, but Ward took him quickly, held him head down, and slapped at his back, urging him to breathe. I could see a pair of little blue balls hanging between his fat thighs, and announced to the unconscious mother and the father standing by her side (he had been given the job of watching her and letting us know should she happen to cease breathing, since we were too tied up with her abdomen to pay much attention to the rest of her) that they were the proud parents of a son. Suddenly this newborn gave out a lusty, room-filling cry. He continued crying vigorously at us from the next room, after Nirma cleaned him up and swaddled him, and kept crying during the entire time that we worked to close up his mom. I'm not usually fond of babies crying, but I have to admit that at that moment, it was a wonderful sound.

Of course we might still lose the mother. There was a dismaying amount of blood. It was probably no more than normal in the circumstances, but it was splashing over the table and down my skirt, the floor was slippery with it, and it was obscuring our field of vision in the abdomen; a loop or two of intestine came surging up from one side. But when I had pushed on the baby's head to dislodge it from the pelvis, it was obvious that Isabel's pelvic girdle was indeed too small. Without the surgery she would have died, and the baby with her. Period. No doubt. None.

I had silently cursed the family's insistence when, way back light-years ago that morning, they had ignored my reassurances that all seemed well and had been determined to accompany me back to my small clinic at the Lodge. Now I praised their instincts, which had turned out to be correct after all.

Still, it's an awful experience to feel out of your depth, in anything. It's especially awful when you're over your head with a human life in your hands. When I laid open the belly of this living person, in miserable light, with no more than semisterile conditions, far from the support of anyone who could aid us if things got even worse than they already were, my heart sank. I wondered whether we would ever be able to make her whole again.

The process of closing the surgical wound, like the rest of this kitchen-table surgery, was less than ideal. Nirma miraculously came up with a few more sterile towels to mop up the blood, but it was still a mess. While I was stitching her incision, Isabel began to recover from the too-small dose of ketamine. A true stoic, she did not move; nonetheless she cried out and kept asking piteously, "What are you doing to me?" My incisions, more or less straight when I'd made them, had somehow become raggedy and crooked without the underlying mass of swollen uterus to stretch the skin. And even before we finished suturing the internal layers together and arrived at the skin, Nirma put down the flashlight with which she'd been illuminating the sutures so that we could see well enough to trim them and began to light the kerosene lamps, signaling that the electricity was about to go off for the night. (Indiana has power only from its own small generating plant, only when it has funds to buy fuel, and even then only from dusk until midnight.)

Nonetheless, we successfully closed one layer after another. The sense of relief as the skin closed over the top of her abdomen was overwhelming.

Just as we peeled off our dripping gloves, the clinic lights blinked out. I used my pocketknife to slice off the plastic nipple on the liter of intravenous fluid we'd brought and started it running into her arm. A blood transfusion would have been better, but that was not an option; at least with the fluid we could boost her circulating volume a bit.

By the time we were finished, it was close to midnight. Arrangements had been made to house Ward and me at the Explorama Inn for what was left of the night, and Nirma agreed to spend the night on duty at the clinic. In the darkness Ward and I walked through the town, then over the slippery jungle path, under a starlit but moonless sky. It takes twenty minutes or so to pass through the town, then another half-hour on narrow paths with several ups and downs to get to the inn. It probably seemed much shorter to me, since I knew the path; I think I said, "only one more hill to go" about ten times. But it was a beautiful starlit night, and although we were both tired, we were still running on adrenaline, so it wasn't at all a bad time to take a hike through the jungle in total darkness.

After arriving at the inn and taking a quick shower, I fell into bed between clean sheets. They felt wonderful. Even my concerns— was she all right? was her son all right? was she hemorrhaging?— faded quickly into exhausted sleep. Our patients were both in Nirma's hands until morning.

Early the next morning, when we returned to the clinic trailed by the TV crew, we found that the baby had been nursing well and was now sleeping peacefully. Isabel winced hard when we touched her incision, but she beamed at us proudly as long as she was allowed to lie still. The CNN people took one look at the as-yet-uncleaned office that had served as our operating room and decided against photographing it. They did take some footage of the happy mother and of me examining her. I have since seen the film and always explain to people that the hysteria that surges through my voice in that footage comes from sheer relief at finding both Isabel and her baby still alive and apparently healthy.

On television, doctors save lives weekly. In real life, there are very few times as a physician when you can say unequivocally that what you did actually "saved a life." This was probably my first, maybe my only, time when there was absolutely no possibility that the patient might have pulled through on her own.

Now that it was all over, and both patients looked healthy, it did feel good.

Still, it had all taken a lot of energy. I felt about five years older, and a little grayer, than I had the day before.

How had I come to be performing operations for which I was entirely unqualified, in the midst of the Amazon rainforest?

The answer begins with my last vacation.

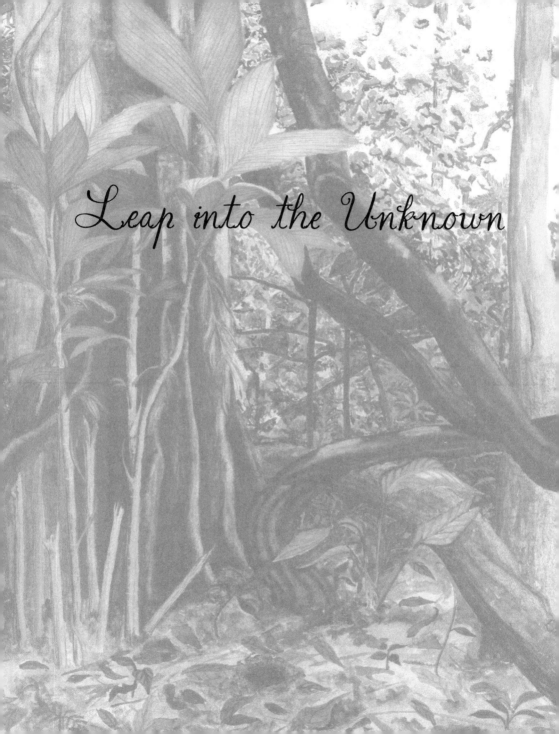

Leap into the Unknown

CHAPTER TWO

# My Last Vacation

In some ways, it isn't at all surprising that I wound up where I did, yet if I had been asked ten years earlier—or one year, or even one week, before my first trip here—I would hardly have predicted that I would soon be deciding to spend years in the Peruvian Amazon.

In 1990 I was a forty-year-old graduate of the University of Wisconsin Medical School with specialty training in internal medicine.

After completing my residency in internal medicine, I joined a small group practice in a town among the rolling hills of west-central Wisconsin. For three years I had been practicing medicine there—and quite happily I might add. I loved my work. My life was full and, for the most part, relaxed. I regularly puttered with my turn-of-the century house and explored the back roads of southwest Wisconsin on my motorcycle.

This was a peaceful time in my life after a decade of studies, and I planned to make it last as long as I could. In fact, up till the time that I left for what turned out to be my last great vacation, if anyone had asked, I would have told them that I would be practicing medicine in Wisconsin until I died, retired, or was sued out of business.

I grew up in Milwaukee, Wisconsin, and was a voracious reader and a good student. College was the obvious next step for me. However, in an attack of impulsiveness, I married at the age of eighteen. The Vietnam War was on, and my new mate went off to join it. When he returned, we moved to Germany for the remaining year of his service. This disrupted the flow of my education, but served to give me a broader view of the world. Germany was hardly uncivilized, yet hot water, for one instance among many, was a luxury not found in every home there, and when it did exist, it usually issued from a small heater perched above bathtub or sink and fed with firewood or coal. This was quite a surprise for someone born and raised in the United States, and it was the first intimation I had of the true wealth of my native country. I have since come to feel that every person born and raised in the U.S. ought to be required to travel abroad, or better yet, make a visit to a less Westernized country, just to see how most of the world lives and to reexamine what is and what is not truly "necessary."

Once we returned home to the United States, my husband and I realized that we had few interests in common. I recovered from my impulsive decision of a few years earlier, and we filed for divorce. Fortunately, he was a good man from whom it was possible to part amicably.

The next few years found me wandering through a series of secretarial jobs, until I landed in The Sunshine Store, a small business that sold exotic houseplants in the small Wisconsin town of Cross Plains. There I also found my true love, Woody.

Unfortunately, love was not enough. Less than a year after we met, he succumbed, abruptly and without much advance warning (at least none that he or I recognized at the time), to a brain tumor, at the age of twenty-four. Devastated, I ran the plant store alone for several years more, then was urged by another friend to return to college for more formal education.

Thus, at the age of twenty-eight, I found myself taking college courses without really knowing where I was heading, only knowing that after so many years, my old interest in learning was being re-kindled. While taking a course in biochemistry with a distinctly applied bent, I decided, quite suddenly and with complete certainty, that I wanted to be a doctor when I grew up.

The next few years were routine, except for my age: I was thirty when I entered medical school. This gave me tremendous freedom; instead of being tied to and hemmed in by grade point averages and semesters, I knew that all of that would end soon enough. I could focus on learning because it was interesting and fun, and that made medical school, and my subsequent residency in internal medicine, interesting and fun, too.

That's how I came to be practicing medicine in Wisconsin a few miles from the house where I had lived for over ten years. Not long after entering practice, I discovered vacations. After years of the rela-tive poverty of studenthood, it suddenly occurred to me that I actu-ally had enough money to afford international trips. The first was to Kenya, where my tour group visited local clinics and were awed by wild animals; the next year it was Egypt, where we visited ancient sites. After those first two trips I was hooked on an annual February escape. I was a member of The Nature Conservancy, and when their magazine showed up with an ad for a trip to the Amazon—"Visit the rain forest! Ride in dugout canoes! See tarantulas and blue morpho butterflies!"—it was too good to pass up. Why not get away from the Wisconsin February blues, go where the temperatures were promised to be in the eighties, and see the original specimens of all my houseplants, in their native habitat, at the same time?

I requested a brochure, which outlined a week at the Explorama ecotourism centers. The Explorama Company, it explained, owns and operates three lodges—Explorama Lodge, the first and still the larg-est and most popular destination; Explorama Inn, the most modern, with indoor plumbing and its own small generating plant, upriver at Indiana; and Explornapo Camp, a more rustic facility, well away from civilization, located in the Sucusari nature preserve, along the Napo River. ACEER (the Amazon Center for Education and Environmental Research) with the associated canopy walkway, a suspension bridge in the treetops, is also within walking distance of Explornapo Camp.

As I was to learn later, the lodges were founded by Peter Jenson, an archaeologist/geologist/anthropologist who came to Peru in the early 1960s to spend two years as one of the first Peace Corps volunteers working at archaeological sites in the Andes.

Having finished his term of service, Peter decided to see the rainforest while he was in the country. He flew to Iquitos, decided to rent a boat and take tourists on day trips down the river, and then founded his own tourist company and settled in for what has turned out to be more than thirty years of operating Explorama Tours.

The Nature Conservancy brochure outlined a week in Explorama's domain, starting with a night at the lodge, moving out to the camp for a couple of nights, then returning to the lodge for the remaining time. It sounded good to me. I signed up to go.

## Saturday, February 10, 1990

The adventure began in Miami. Having left Wisconsin in snow, I arrived in Miami around dusk, stepped out into warm humid air, and began sweating. I could feel the crick in my neck melting already, after having plagued me for the last three days before departure. I already felt like I was on vacation. The clinic and hospital and beepers all seemed far behind.

The plane to Iquitos, Peru, wasn't leaving till 8:00 P.M., but we were supposed to congregate two hours ahead of time at the Faucett Airlines departure counter, so about 5:00 P.M. I started heading in that direction. I strolled at a leisurely pace to the place where I was supposed to meet the tour group. No one was there yet.

Then, suddenly, a harried-looking man ran over, peered at my baggage tag, looked up my name on the clipboard he carried, and dashed me over to the check-in counter, explaining that the departure time had been moved up two hours and the plane was to leave in fifteen minutes! We ran, not walked, to our gate at the far end of the concourse, frantically hoping that the plane had not left us behind.

On our breathless arrival, however, passengers and baggage alike were scattered over the floor. We were told that an engine was being serviced and we wouldn't leave until 9:30 P.M. That was OK with me. They could take all the time they wanted. I was on vacation, in no hurry to do anything, and I wanted them to get it right before I got on that plane.

We finally boarded at 11:00 P.M., three hours late—my first encounter with the South American sense of scheduling. When we touched down on the Iquitos runway, a round of applause went up from the Peruvian passengers, and a missionary sitting next to me expressed surprise . . . he explained that more often than not, the plane wouldn't bother to stop at Iquitos, but would continue straight on to Lima (where the pilots lived and their girlfriends were waiting), from whence the Iquitos-bound passengers would be ferried back the following morning. We checked into our hotel in Iquitos at 6:00 A.M., in time to get ninety minutes of sleep before boarding a bus that took us to the launch for our two-and-a-half-hour trip down the Amazon to Explorama Lodge.

### Sunday, February 11

And an interesting trip it was. At Iquitos, the Amazon is over two miles wide and up to one hundred feet deep. Its mouth is 2,300 miles away, on the east coast of South America, but oceangoing freight ships power their way all the way upriver to this major inland port. The water is light brown and opaque, filled with silt from the banks that crumble constantly into the river, sometimes even as we watched. Although the surface of the water is smooth, even sometimes glassy, the current surges along at a brisk four miles per hour, with immense force.

The boat that brought us to the lodge was low and long, with benches along both sides, low walls, and a thatched roof whose ridgepole ran the length of the boat. The steersman sat up in front, and in back was an outboard motor running on gasoline siphoned from an open fifty-gallon drum. Behind the motor was the outdoor restroom overhanging the water (offerings from what one wag had christened "the poop deck" simply dropped into the river). I eagerly photographed several of the colorful boats passing us, filled with local people, chickens, and big bunches of bananas, then realized that our boat looked just the same, minus the produce. We were traveling just like the locals.

The twenty-one people on our trip settled in. Some napped; most stared eagerly at the sights of the forest and river. Everyone was drenched with sweat, even at this early hour. It was not only warm; it was humid—a weather condition that I soon learned spanned all seasons.

We were delivered by boat directly to the lodge because it was high-water season; in the dry months, we were told, it is a fifteen-minute walk in from the river. We were greeted at the Bar Tahuampa ("The Swamp") by a nice young man with a tray of what turned out to be glasses filled with sugarcane rum and Inca Kola. This latter is a bubble-gum-flavored, yellow, syrupy soft drink endemic to Peru, not very palatable by itself (at least to *gringos*) but quite seductive when diluted with the locally made rum.

Our rooms were all connected by thatch-roofed walkways. The rooms had no doorknobs, locks, or latches, but they did have hooks on the outside to hold the door shut when you were out and hooks inside to hold it shut when you were in. There was a kerosene lantern in each room, more lanterns sat on small shelves built into the hallway walls, and little metal lamps that looked like miniature smudge pots lined the pathways. Each room had two beds, each securely enclosed by a mosquito net, as well as a couple of hooks, towels and hangers, a small set of shelves for clothes and gear, and a table with a basin and big pitcher of wash water. After washing, we were instructed just to toss the water out the back window, which had neither glass nor screen, just a waist-high wall with a curtain above—totally open to the jungle.

In a separate shower hut, each shower was an enclosure with walls of wild cane, which resembles bamboo, with a bench along one side and a big flat showerhead from which poured a limitless quantity of cool water. The latrines had dirt floors, comfortable seats, and none of the smell I recalled from my Girl Scout outings. The atmosphere of the whole place was rustic but quite comfortable.

After lunch, I retired to a hammock on one of the patios and snoozed away the effects of the rum and cola. Then we split into two groups, one guided by Roldan and the other by Lucio, and we went on our first jungle walk.

The paths were red clay mud, ankle-deep in many places, though stepping-logs had been laid out along most of the way. We weren't even out of the camp yet, pausing while Roldan pointed out the site of the original Explorama Lodge (moved to higher ground because it flooded too often), when I felt first one, then another, then a flurry of tiny but intense stings around my ankles. "Fire ants!" They were tiny and red and ferocious, but fortunately they could be brushed off and squished and didn't seem to inflict any lasting damage. Still, it was my first lesson in jungle walking: look before you put any body part anywhere, including standing still!

Ants abound in rain forests. Besides the fire ants, we saw army ants, busy columns of red ants three-eighths of an inch long, bustling rapidly across our path in perpetual motion, disappearing into the jungle on their unknown missions. And there were parasol (leafcutter) ants, small black critters carrying pieces of leaves over their heads, ferrying them in a fire-brigade line back to their nest, where they pile them up and cultivate an edible (for them) fungus. Roldan scared up a poison ant, a black monster an inch-and-a-quarter long, with hind-quarters like a wasp's, and informed us that the poison ants are one of the sources of curare, as well as being famous for the intensity of the pain they inflict with their bite.

We saw a tarantula, brown and gray and furry. One of the group spotted him lurking in a big bromeliad beside the path, and Roldan took the bromeliad apart leaf by leaf (cautiously). Each time the spider tried to scurry for cover Roldan pulled the cover away, until finally the poor creature gave up and sat still on the forest path for us to coo over and photograph at leisure.

Huge, iridescent blue morpho butterflies floated through the air, as well as smaller ones of assorted colors and shapes, many of them brilliantly hued, others transparent as glass. Someone spotted a millipede, easily three inches long, which Roldan picked up to show us that it was harmless. I let it crawl on my hand, and it tickled. These crawlers have precise rectangular segments that make them look as though they are manufactured instead of hatched. The group with Lucio spotted a sloth, but the best we could do for mammalian life was a swinging vine where Roldan assured us a marmoset had been, moments before.

The bird-watchers went nuts—there was such variety.

And of course the plants were spectacular. There were spathiphyllums and gingers and podocarpuses and pothos and philodendrons and bananas and heliconias, and plants I recognized but couldn't recall the names of, and others I didn't even recognize. There were mahogany trees and ceiba trees and ficus trees with huge draped buttress roots. Some were crosshatched with scars where the local people had cut them for the sap, which they drink as a cure for intestinal parasites.

One of the ficuses had buttresses at its base extending at least thirty feet in each direction. A liana hung from its branches (fifty or sixty feet above the forest floor, and those were just the lower branches), and we all played Tarzan. The vine had a surprising amount of give to it, but you could get the feel of swinging on it pretty easily. The only thing was, when you went flying back to the tree, you had to remember to put your feet out to keep you from bashing into the trunk, which loomed more like a wall than a tree.

After returning to camp, several of us took a swim. All the best travel authorities advise against such activities, but the guides said it was OK, so we jumped off the boat dock into the warm muddy waters, and it was wonderful.

**Monday, February 12**
Rain came down in torrents the first night, but I slept blissfully through it. The next morning, the sky was gray and drippy and the red clay paths were mud. We piled back into the covered boat and headed down the Amazon, hung a left at the Napo River, and went two more hours up the Napo to reach the Sucusari Stream and Napo Camp. Along the way, freshwater dolphins cavorted.

In the afternoon, we again went for a long jungle walk. At Napo, the forest floor had more humus, with lots of fallen leaves. If you didn't look up into the canopy and didn't try to actually identify the plants, it could almost have passed for a temperate forest. Almost.

Lucio, our guide for the day, whose grandfather was a *brujo* (a shaman, or medicine man), pointed out many medicinal plants. There was one that he said is used for birth control. For this purpose, he explained, the sap is mixed with rum (an indispensable ingredient in many *brujo* brews) and sugar and left to ferment for three months. A woman drinks one shot glass of the concoction each morning before breakfast, for two weeks beginning just after her menses, and she becomes sterile, without any change in her menstrual periods. I wished I knew the physiology of that one.

We also saw a slender tree with a white surface that was a fungus, like the chalky coating on Brie cheese, that fluoresces at night after rain. And we saw trees whose sap was reported to stop diarrhea, cure constipation, poison the intestinal parasites endemic to this place, and combat anemia—more amazing by the minute.

After dinner that night, we went out in the open boats. The sides were low, with board seats along the top edge (don't lean back!). When we boarded, on the floor was a turtle called a "Matamata," with a bizarre head that perfectly resembled a dry leaf. The variety and general weirdness of the Amazonian fauna (and flora, too) is astonishing.

We floated from the Sucusari Stream to the Napo River and found a caiman, an anaconda, and a kinkajou.

The caiman (an alligator relative) was a young one, maybe six months old according to Lucio, who by leaning precariously over the front of the boat caught it by the tail and behind the head and carried it around for all of us to see. It was two or three feet long, with skin like an alligator's and a long snout full of very sharp, thin teeth. The caiman was mad, too, and hissed at us the whole time. When Lucio threw it back, he made sure to give it a good toss and to keep his hands well out of the way of the angry mouth.

The anaconda was coiled on a dead branch sticking out of the water, tasting the night air with its tongue. Since Lucio had gotten the caiman, Roldan volunteered to catch the anaconda, which was three or four feet long. The only problem was that our spotlight attracted an assortment of insects, including some night-flying wasps, and Roldan was stung several times. He held onto the snake, however, and we all petted it cautiously before he turned it loose to slither away on the surface of the water.

The kinkajou, a little monkeylike creature, was playing high in the branches of a tall tree. Returning along the Sucusari Stream, we also saw a porcupine on another tree trunk, and in the topmost branches of the tallest tree, eighty or a hundred feet above our heads, a big brown furry sloth.

## Tuesday, February 13

The next day, we arose before dawn to go bird-watching. For me it was also an excuse for a dawn boat ride. It was a beautiful time to be out, with steam rising off the river's surface, local people moving about and fishing, and their cooking fires sending up trails of fragrant smoke. I have since come to love this time of day, and even in that first week long ago, I was intrigued by the realities of a life which begins at dawn and closes down at sunset and in which fire must be kindled before breakfast can be prepared.

After our breakfast, cooked over an open hearth like the ones used by the locals, we went up a small tributary of the Napo as far as we could in open boats. When the vegetation closed in so that the boat could go no further, we disembarked and marched through the jungle for half an hour to an oxbow lake with black, clear, deep water. Dugout canoes were tethered where the footpath ended, and with only a little trepidation, we got into the low-riding primitive craft, careful not to wiggle much (or else water came in over the edge), and were paddled around the lake. There were *Victoria amazonia* water lilies, four feet across, and birds and bats clinging to the underside of a fallen tree. The bats looked like bits of dried mud until, startled by our approach, they took flight.

By midday, the sun was fully out, and the insects were buzzing by. The afternoon's activities were a nap in the hammock, then a visit to a *ribereño* (river people) village. One of the inhabitants was the supervisor at the camp, who let us just wander through his home. Unlike the Africans and Egyptians, who in my experience either didn't want to be photographed or else wanted to be paid for it, the people here seemed to enjoy the attention and smiled shyly for us. In one house they gave us *chicha*, a fermented corn drink, very much like thin creamed corn with vodka percolating up through—awful, actually, but worth trying for the experience.

After returning again to camp and sizing up the extent of the day's sunburn, several of us went swimming in the stream, off the dock. A piranha had been caught there the day before, but Lucio assured us that piranhas don't really eat you alive (at least not as long as you're not bleeding), so we jumped in and splashed around, and sure enough, no one got eaten.

That night after dark we motored far up the Sucusari. The sky was clear and filled with unfamiliar stars. I recognized Orion and the Pleiades, but that was it. For North Americans, of course, the Peruvian sky looked upside down. The change in perspective was startling.

After going upstream, we turned off the motor and drifted silently down. At least we were silent. The forest was filled with the sounds of katydids and frogs and birds and the occasional splash of something sliding off a log into the murky water. It was magical, we all agreed.

There was even a shooting star.

**Wednesday, February 14**
On Wednesday, there were the usual predawn rain showers; then I laid awake listening to jungle noises. My watch claimed it was almost 6:30, so I got up as quietly as I could, went out to the dining area, and since no one was around, went down to the dock and sat and watched the bats catching mosquitoes.

Eventually, as I sat there, the bats were replaced by butterflies. Daylight began to filter through the clouds, and I started to see water-skimmer bugs dashing across the surface of the stream. Every now and again, there would be a bigger-than-waterbug splash. The calls in the jungle changed as night was slowly replaced by day. It was a lovely, peaceful early morning, with smells, sounds, sights, and atmosphere all quite far removed from what I was so well accustomed to back home. The tranquility was magical.

My ruminations concluded at breakfast. After breakfast we motored out to the Napo River and into a creek in the middle of the island. We floated past huge mangrove trees with roots hanging down into the water. We saw a three-toed sloth and many birds, including a pair of blue-crowned trogons. These are parrot-sized birds with cobalt blue on their heads, wings, and backs and flame red on their chests. We stopped to pick some fragrant white flowers that were weighing down a huge bush overhanging the stream.

Finally we parked beneath the biggest mangrove we could find. Roldan cut up pieces of raw beef and baited hooks on poles made of straight, thin, debarked branches. Then we all went fishing. We caught one piranha and several catfish. While we were fishing, a troop of saddle-back tamarin monkeys came clambering across the creek from a small tree on the far side into our mangrove and frolicked above us. Back at Napo Camp, we had the piranha and catfish for lunch.

Then a long boat ride, four or five hours in the thatched-roof boat, out the Sucusari, down the Napo, and up the Amazon, back to Explorama Lodge in time for another swim, a little laundry, a shower, and an adjournment to the Bar Tahuampa, where I was not even halfway through a rum and Inca Kola before losing motivation for journal writing. But had I been able to see into my own subconscious, I would have had to write "Oops . . . neither Kenya nor Egypt felt quite like this. This place is starting to seep into my blood. Where did you say home was?"

**Thursday, February 15, before breakfast at the lodge**
Thursday, I was up again before dawn, and the moon was directly overhead, reflecting on the water beneath the bridge.

The river seemed high already, but it was still rising, and rapidly. It was clear that here during high-water season, everything not on stilts would be submerged.

After breakfast, we crossed the river and parked up a side stream on the other side of the Amazon. Some of us went fishing for piranha from the open boat, and some of us went swimming from the other side of the same boat. We had quizzed Lucio and Roldan numerous times about the advisability of this arrangement, and they had assured us, "no problem." After I had proven luckless as an angler (and after Roldan had jumped in first, fishing pole in hand), I dove in.

The secret to catching piranhas, we discovered, is to have a long line (because they hover near the bottom) and to splash the water with the end of your pole so they think something has fallen in (which obviously brings to mind questions regarding the wisdom of our swimming arrangements). Of course, you use red meat for bait. A little blood also helps. After a long dry spell, Lucio finally pulled one in. As he took it off the hook, the ungrateful thing bit him viciously. He then smeared the blood from his thumb on his next piece of bait and quickly hooked another, then another, and another, twelve or fifteen in all.

Between piranha fishing, swimming in the Amazon (well, one of its tributaries), lunch of cold chicken and potatoes and cucumber slices and hearts of palm drizzled with lime juice, napping on the shaded seats of the thatch boat, and swimming off its bow, we could hardly have asked for a better picnic or a more relaxed day.

### Friday, February 16, at the lodge

On Friday, February 16, I awoke at dawn, with the half moon directly above. I walked out and sat on the dock for the last morning of this vacation. I wasn't sure I wanted to go home. I was not alone in that feeling; our group had talked about it in the bar the night before, and we were unanimously in despair that this was to be our last day. Again, however, had I been able to consult my subconscious—and amazingly, it was, even then, still subconscious—I would have realized that my reluctance to leave stemmed from more than the usual feelings that everyone experiences at the close of an especially satisfying vacation.

After breakfast we walked the "Bushmaster," the most arduous of the lodge's jungle trails. By midmorning the temperature rose to ninety degrees, with humidity so high that it felt as though we were walking through mist. Our guide explained that the bushmaster is a snake in the rattlesnake family: up to twelve feet long, highly poisonous, and much feared. The trail is so named because of the many snakes encountered while it was being cut. Fortunately, we saw no snakes and returned safely home for a rest before lunch.

I was just relaxing again when I heard the thunder of feet along the boardwalk and heard someone shout, "She's in Room 40!" and then, "She's not here!" I tumbled quickly out of the mosquito net and contradicted him.

The commotion was centered at the guides' house at the far end of the lodge. It seemed that one of the lodge's workers had been bitten by a fer-de-lance, a smaller, but still deadly, relative of the bushmaster. The man had been cutting grass with a machete and had surprised the snake when he reached under the log where it was snoozing. The lodge possessed antivenin (two years past its expiration date, but probably still good), but someone was needed to administer it. When I arrived, the patient looked calm but worried, with a piece of string tied loosely above his ankle. Despite the tourniquet, his foot was already red and swollen. While fifteen or twenty of the other employees and guides sat quietly around, lending support and contributing atmosphere, I popped the cap off the antivenin. It was a white powder in a small vial, requiring only sterile water to reconstitute it. I drew the water into the syringe, injected it into the vial, and shook furiously (the vial, not me personally). Normally, one is supposed to administer a test dose of plain horse serum, because some people react violently, even fatally, to the antivenin. However, the test dose was in absentia, and since the patient was already numb up to the thigh, it seemed worth the risk to give the stuff.

Another shoestring was produced and tied above his elbow while I upended the syringe and tapped out the air bubbles. Everyone was anxious and silent as I inserted the needle into his antecubital vein. The antivenin went in as I divided my attention between the slowly emptying syringe and the young man's face. Then I removed the make-shift tourniquet. There was no stethoscope, but by using a toilet paper tube as a crude substitute, I could hear a normal heartbeat and clear lungs. He was later taken by motorboat to the city, where he eventually recovered completely.

I, however, did not recover. I already knew that I wasn't ready for the trip to end, but it still hadn't quite hit me fully. During the week I'd made friends with Pam, the key Explorama staffer at the lodge, and she had told me her story. Pam is a former high school science teacher from Connecticut who got to wondering how it was that the art teachers got to go to Europe with their students, while the science teachers didn't go anywhere except the lab. She began to arrange a few trips for her students, one of which brought them, and her, to the Amazon and to Explorama Lodge. She was so intrigued by the place that she later returned to do some research for her master's degree; as she tells it, she met Peter Jenson at the airport, where he offered her a job for the summer. Being a teacher, she had the summer free, so she accepted. By the time of my trip there in 1990, she had been in the country working with Explorama for more than five years and had recently married one of the Explorama guides. Since this was a summer job, however, she swears that she will go home as soon as the first snow falls.

After the diversion with the snakebite, I gave her my address and mentioned that I would be open to the idea of coming down to serve as the lodge doctor every now and then, should Explorama have such a need. Of course, I said, I couldn't leave my practice in Wisconsin, but I thought I could get away for a few weeks or a month periodically...

However, somewhere in between midday Friday and 3:00 A.M. Saturday, the assigned hour for getting up (arise at 3:00 A.M., breakfast at 3:30, leave the Lodge at 4:00 for the four-hour trip back up to the city and points beyond), my eccentric streak exerted itself seriously. When I woke at 2:30 and took a last cup of coffee to the bridge outside the dining room, I found myself looking at a night sky filled with fireflies and lightning and thinking that if I had to leave this place, I would shrivel up and expire. I didn't even want to go to the historic ancient city of Cuzco, thinking superstitiously that once I left Explorama, I would never be able to get back. I told myself that this was an absurd idea, that it would be far too costly to stay at the lodge as a single tourist, that the Cuzco trip would undoubtedly be fascinating (and it was), that I didn't speak Spanish beyond my three-word vocabulary, that there was no support system for a physician here—no professional backup, no laboratory or x-ray or pharmacy, not even a place in which to work— that I had a wonderful practice back in Wisconsin, not to mention a wonderful home where I had lived for nearly thirteen years. I told myself all of this, but none of it made any impression on my subconscious, which was now becoming conscious. I didn't want to leave. I couldn't leave.

I negotiated a compromise with myself: OK, how about this— I'll go to Cuzco, do all the things I am supposed to do as a tourist, and go home, all as scheduled. Then I will see how I feel once I am home again, back in familiar surroundings.

However, once I reached home, it failed to feel any longer like home. My instinct still said, "Peru, Peru, Peru…" This feeling must seem rather strange to anyone who has not experienced it. You'd think that I would reflect on the decision, figure out various options, and make a thorough plan. But I didn't. Like falling in love with Woody, or deciding to go to medical school, the decision to return to the jungle, as irrational as it may seem, just sort of jumped out at me fully grown. It was that clear and that sudden. What can I say? I seem to be an impulsive kind of person.

Pam and Peter offered to provide me with one of the lodge's guest rooms in which to offer medical services to local people as well as to be on call for Explorama's guests. Without hesitation I agreed to do just that for three months.

So it was that in May of 1990, armed with the contents of a doctor's "black bag," one bottle of prenatal vitamins, a small microscope, and a three-month leave of absence from my Wisconsin practice, I returned to Peru. Certainly once I was here, I would come to my senses, find that the magic of the forest was not quite so compelling once I was actually living in it. Then I would go back to the life of a normal physician, in a normal practice, in a normal country.

Well, that's what I told myself.

# CHAPTER THREE

# Setting Up Shop

There was no certainty that setting up a medical practice in Peru would work out. In fact, from the perspective of any typical U.S. middle-class standard, it was highly unlikely that I would achieve anything more than getting bitten by a few mosquitos (if not worse). And, from a financial point of view, moving from a Wisconsin medical practice to the middle of the jungle was unquestionably economic suicide—at the least. One of my partners at the clinic at home shook his head and said frankly, "You're crazy, Linnea."

I didn't leave my native land lightly. Even more worrying than the monetary costs were the personal ones. All I had to go on was my crazy intuition that it was absolutely imperative to my sanity that I go live in that jungle—not much to put into the balance against the departure from friends, family, language, culture, and ice cream whenever I felt like it.

Nonetheless, the intuition was irresistible, so, doubts or no, I continued packing up my life. On the day before I left, I rode my motorcycle through the beautiful rolling hills of southwest Wisconsin and recalled the words of a farmer neighbor of mine (the architect of Stonehedge, a wonderful collection of primitive stone and glass sculpture), who claimed, "If a person can't be happy on a small farm in Wisconsin, he doesn't have the makings of happiness in his heart." I had been happy these years in Wisconsin. And yet, ever since that February week in the jungle, that faraway and still mostly unknown place had beckoned me to make it home.

I was going, at any rate. If my intuition proved to be faulty, as I more than half expected would be the case, at least I was only committed to three months' time.

As I left for Peru on June 2, 1990, I retraced my steps of four months before, but in a very different frame of mind. I was delighted, relieved, and apprehensive all at once, and could hardly comprehend that I was actually going to work, not vacation. The plane from Miami to Iquitos actually landed in Iquitos, which in those days happened only about half the time. I sailed straight through customs with no questions asked and spent a short night in the tourist hotel *(Las Turistas)* before waking to pouring rain for my first day of life in the Amazon basin. Here I was, crossing my own personal Rubicon—only in this case it was the mother of all rivers, the Amazon.

After breakfast, I went to Explorama's office/garage/boat dock/headquarters to board the *pamacari* (thatch-roof boat) that took me, in two-and-a-half hours, to the lodge at Yanamono. I tried to be cool on the trip downriver, but I was bubbling over inside at being here once again, with nary a doubt as to the wisdom of having pulled up my roots of the last four decades.

On arrival at Explorama Lodge, my new home-to-be, I was shown to room number 2, just past the dining room. It was as close as one could get to what was to be my new clinic, and in a location where a call in the middle of the night would disrupt no more than a few sleeping tourists.

I unfolded my clothes and unpacked my toothbrush, notebooks, insect repellent, shoes, and shampoo. I put the medical equipment into a basket left over from a long-ago trip to the Bahamas and now transported to an even more exotic part of the world.

Then I walked bravely down the steps of the long house in which my room was located, across twenty feet of packed-dirt path, up the next steps, and along the walkway in front of the *comedor* (dining room), across the thatch-roofed wooden bridge over the now almost dry stream, down the stairs at the far side, along another fifty feet of packed dirt parallel to the house where the guides sleep, and up the stairs into an open area at the end of the guides' dormitory.

The house is around thirty feet wide by seventy or eighty feet long, built on pilings about four feet tall, to keep the floor above the annual floods. The periphery of the building is a half-wall of overlapping planks, and there is a completely unwalled area at one end, the *sala* (living room). The roof is palm thatch. A central corridor runs lengthwise, with rooms opening off either side. The new clinic was the last room on the north side, sharing a wall with the *sala*, which was about to become the waiting room for my embryonic clinic.

The clinic itself had been, until the previous night, a sleeping room for one of the guides. He had been unceremoniously rousted and moved down the hall, and his quarters were presented to me. The room measured nine by twelve feet, with plywood walls, no ceiling, and the outer half-wall facing the Bar Tahuampa. In the open space above the half-wall hung a curtain, heavy with smoke from the kerosene lamps. A kerosene lamp still occupied a small shelf, and a pitcher and basin of ceramic-glazed iron were placed on a small stool to serve as my water supply and sink.

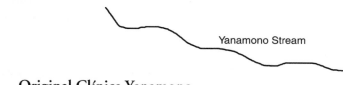

## Original Clínica Yanamono

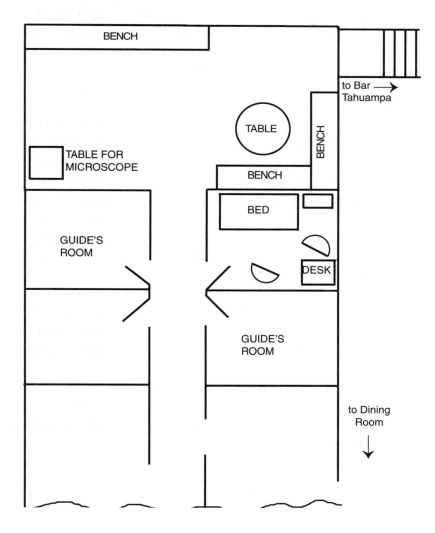

In Wisconsin, I had worked in a clinic with running water, electric lights, built-in laboratory, and x-ray suite; a small but well-equipped hospital next door for really ill patients; as many nurses, aides, and other helping hands as I could want; a community of doctors of various specialties to call on for advice and/or assistance (with ready means by which to make such calls); and MedFlight ready at a moment's notice to transfer critically ill patients to the tertiary care facilities of the University Hospital in Madison, where I'd trained. What was here wasn't exactly what I had left behind, but it was what I had to work with now.

Before departing from Wisconsin, I had agonized at length over what I could or should bring. Pam had warned me about customs (*aduana*)—no rules except theirs; anything medicinal and/or high-technological was fair game for seizure ("decommissioning," they call it), with no easy way, or sometimes no way at all, to recover items once they'd been confiscated. Besides, the airline limited me to two suitcases (although at the time I didn't realize just how weighty they could be) and a carry-on. Should I try to take everything with me and risk losing it all at customs in the Iquitos airport? Or take a minimum and risk trying to find what I needed in Iquitos, where I could already anticipate a Third World infrastructure?

Decisions, decisions.

I finally settled on the most vital tools and a few extras. Into my two suitcases went my stethoscope, oto-ophthalmoscope (a glorified flashlight used to look into eyes, ears, and throats), and a blood-pressure cuff. This was more or less the equivalent of the carpenter's hammer, saw, and measuring tape, without the additional refinements of, say, file or rasp, level, sawhorse, or T-square, to say nothing of power saws or electric drills. Most medicines (nails and lumber) would also have to be obtained in the new locale.

In the basement of my Wisconsin clinic I had unearthed a big box of prenatal vitamins, outdated and therefore destined in the

U.S. for the trash, but probably still effective. Cathy, our clinic nurse, had cheerfully volunteered an hour or two of her time, and we sat cross-legged on the basement floor, ripping open packets of one or two tablets each and dumping the vitamins into a plastic jar. While in the basement, I noticed a small black microscope sitting high up on a shelf. It used a mirror instead of the electric light that is universally employed today, and turned out to belong to Dusty Koch, one of my partners, being a relic of his medical school days. He graciously gave permission for me to take it, so it also entered my suitcase (and small though it was, it was surprisingly heavy). I bought a few dozen tablets of two or three different antibiotics to round out my medicine supply. Lastly, I included a couple of books—the PDR (Physician's Desk Reference), which contains trade and generic names, uses, doses, contraindications (reasons not to use a medicine in a particular patient or situation), and side effects of thousands of medicines; a small general medical reference; and a tiny looseleaf notebook in which I had accumulated ten years' worth of "pearls," the abbreviated but highly valued nuggets of fact, opinion, comparison, and miscellany, handed from attending physicians to residents, residents to interns, interns to students. Over the years, the self-evident, superfluous, and already well-memorized items had gradually been weeded out, and what remained was, for me, a reference library in miniature. I also included a small paperback book on gynecology and obstetrics, because I knew I'd be seeing at least some OB, and I had virtually no training or experience in that field outside of what I'd picked up as a student.

Those were my supplies, the substitute for all I had left in high-tech, fully equipped Wisconsin. One small armload of books and tools, and what was lodged in my cerebrum, was my entire stock in trade.

I set my small armload on the table in the *sala*. This table was no more than a six-inch-thick crosswise slice of some rain-forest tree, balanced on a supporting frame of two-by-fours. I stood back, took a photograph, and laughed at myself, half in amazement, half in despair.

People sometimes ask if I have ever panicked and regretted my decision to come here, and I have to admit that during these first few moments of setting up the new "clinic," I came pretty close. That was when the realization of what I was doing hit me the hardest. I had just left my house, my friends, my family, my country, and all the services, equipment, machinery, and other adjuncts of modern medicine in the developed world, in order to come to this strange new place where I didn't even speak the language. When I unpacked the very few, very basic instruments I had brought and put them into the raggedy basket along with the minuscule collection of books and meager stock of medicines I had with me, it all made a distressingly small bundle in my arms. As I had walked from my room past the dining hall and along the path to the site of what was to be my new clinic, it seemed as though I was walking a very long way from Wisconsin. And when I set my things down on that sawed-off log in the large and very empty open area that was the guides' living room and soon to become my patients' waiting room, the contrast between the smallness of my collection of tools, and the vastness of the space, both literal and figurative, in which they were set, was rather daunting. My thought, actually, was "Ohmygod, what do I think I am doing?"

Probably, under the circumstances, it was a most appropriate question.

Pam came along to help me move in. While I ruminated on the wisdom of my recent decision, she was busy flicking cobwebs and squashed bugs from the walls with a towel. Orlando, one of the room boys, came and helped move the bed around and carried in an open bookcase; César, the administrator of the lodge, who had evidently once served as some sort of medic, came and supervised shyly, then vanished, only to reappear some time later with a newly resurfaced small table for the little microscope. I sorted out the few medicines I'd brought, made a sketch, at Pam's suggestion, for a proposed cabinet to hold them, and gave the sketch to César. Temporarily the meds would occupy the bookshelf, along with the books and instruments.

Later, I came back, only to find Orlando taking the bed apart and cleaning each of its wooden slats, resweeping the floor, and spiffing up the curtain. I apparently had a most eager and helpful new "staff."

I had fretted a bit, wondering who would be my first patient. I spoke almost no Spanish. Pam had offered to translate for me, but what if Pam was not around? I conjured up images of a patient in serious need of immediate treatment, with her relatives all talking at me in rapid-fire Spanish, while I futilely flipped through my dictionary trying to translate.

As it happened, the morning after my arrival I had my first patient. As I walked back to the clinic end of the lodge, there was a sweet, shy, and very nervous girl, ten years old and looking eight (her grandmother who had brought her looked fifty but was probably my age). Grandma explained; Ary, one of the Explorama guides, translated for me; Melina Gisela, the patient, listened meekly; and I asked questions through Ary, trying to catch as much as I could of Grandma's answers while smiling reassuringly at my patient. When I brought her back from the waiting room where we'd been talking to the exam room now designated "clinic," I am sure she was thoroughly terrified. But she gave no sign of it and followed me obediently while Grandma waited on the verandah. She'd had two weeks of abdominal pain, with cramping and bloody diarrhea. The girl was not acutely ill, had good bowel sounds, and as I palpated her tiny abdomen, evidenced only a little pain in the left lower quadrant (well away from the appendix, which would have worried me), without any masses or organomegaly (enlargement of liver or spleen, which would have signified serious illness).

I had not yet learned to ask whether the family was drinking their river water raw, as most families do, or boiling it first, but the history and exam were both consistent with an amoebic infection. I went for my stash of metronidazole and measured out the necessary dose, cutting adult-sized tablets in half for this fragile child. I was hoping I was right about its being amoebae, because I had no medicine yet for intestinal worms, and besides, on my first patient I wanted to be right. Stool analysis would have been nice, but that was among the many luxuries I had left behind in Wisconsin. Thus, I was delighted when Grandma said the equivalent of "Ah, that's why all the worm medicine I've been dosing her with hasn't worked."

So, my first patient would be a success—at least, if she took the medicine as prescribed, and if it worked as it should, and if I hadn't missed some other obvious or obscure diagnostic possibility.

Word of my arrival spread rapidly via the grapevine, which although not always accurate is invariably active. Within days I began to see a steady trickle of patients. As with most medical practices, the majority had common and quite treatable problems—worms, cuts, colds, diarrhea, stomach pains, toothaches, skin problems, pneumonia, and bronchitis. All of these ailments, some more serious than others, are easily treated, so long as you understand what the patient is telling you, you make the right diagnosis, and you have the right medicines.

As to the first need—understanding the patient—Pam was a constant companion and a godsend for me. (The guides also helped with translation, but they came and went on erratic schedules, and they were men, reluctant to translate for a woman with any sort of "female problems." In this culture, men do not inquire too closely regarding any of the functions of female bodies, not even of their own wives.) The first year or two here, I would not have been able to make it without Pam. She translated for me until I learned enough to do it myself, she helped me to be accepted at

Explorama, she kept me company in the jungle (she was living at the lodge in those days), and she was just generally a friend. She now lives in the city, but remains my best friend in Peru, sharing her family with me and providing a sounding board for ideas and a home for me when I visit the city. She remains a teacher at heart, having developed (along with Lee Peavy of International Expeditions) the Adopt-A-School program that uses donations from tourists to provide school supplies for a couple dozen schools along the river.

Pam is a gem. And in the beginning, she kept the communication going smoothly.

As far as the second requirement—making the correct diagnosis—I seemed to be doing pretty well, considering the lack of diagnostic equipment and options. Most of my patients were getting better fairly quickly. Fortunately, I had not yet been confronted with any critically ill patients, although they would sooner or later come, I was sure.

Regarding that third essential—having the right medicines— the small stock that I had brought with me was being rapidly depleted. I needed to go shopping in Iquitos.

Thus it was that I rose at predawn one Saturday to catch the boat making the three-and-a-half-hour trip upriver to the city ( in the local "river taxis," it can be as much as eight or nine hours, so I wasn't about to complain). Pam went with me. After two weeks of being at the lodge, she had a free day or two to spend in the city with her husband and family. We were treated to a gorgeous peach-colored dawn breaking on the river behind us as we slowly moved upriver.

A couple of days earlier, Pam had taken me upriver to the Explorama Inn at Indiana and had provided lunch so that I could grill an RN who was working at the Indiana clinic, in order to prioritize my pharmaceutical "shopping list." I'd asked her, "What are the most common illnesses here? With what medicines are they customarily treated? Is there a program for people with tuberculosis? What about family planning?" and on and on. Armed with her answers, Pam and I descended upon the city, looking to trade money for medicine.

Even though it is cut off from the outside world, Iquitos is the hub of the rainforest area of Peru, the only metropolis in this entire quarter of the country. It has grown from a town of about five thousand in the early 1960s to somewhere near half a million now, if you count the thousands living in the dirt-floored shacks of the *pueblos jovenes* (young towns)—the term "slums" having been officially outlawed by one of the previous governments. The center of the city is a dozen blocks of commercial district that is paved; the rest of the streets are just dirt, dusty and uneven on dry days and a sea of mud when it rains.

It is an immensely poor, intensely populated area. There is one part of the city sometimes optimistically called "the Venice of the Amazon," where the poor houses are built on rafts instead of on the usual stilts. They used to float in the filthy water of the Río Itaya where it flows into the Amazon. Unfortunately, the Itaya has changed its course, so many of the shacks are now floating on mud flats, especially in the low-water season. The poverty is stunning; suffice it to say, you wouldn't want to live there if you're committed to U.S. living standards.

Once we arrived in Iquitos, the question was, where do we go now to find a wholesale pharmacy? Fortunately, we ran into Edgard, another of the seemingly ubiquitous Explorama guides, who promptly, cheerfully, and unquestioningly commandeered the Explorama minivan with which to gallantly escort us. We were directed to two pharmacies, but both were low on inventory. However, the fellow manning the counter at the last place sent us around the corner to the Plaza de Armas (Military Square), and there we struck gold.

Every Central or South American town has a *Plaza de Armas*, with monuments to the heroes of all the wars that have been lost. In

Iquitos, the buildings around the plaza date from the rubber boom at the turn of the century. It was to one of these formerly elegant, now decaying, structures that we were directed.

The building was probably constructed as some sort of mercantile center, with living quarters upstairs. By the time we arrived, ninety years later, the ground floor was what was called a pharmacy, though it displayed more shampoo, clothespins, and frying pans than medicines. Upstairs, however, we discovered what turned out to be a wholesale drug warehouse. Eureka!

This warehouse was well stocked with antibiotics, and we went on a spree. We were given permission to roam through the shelves, shaking dust off yellowing cardboard boxes, and were amazed at some of the items they were selling—Lopid, for example, used to treat high cholesterol, when with the diet most people consume here, there probably isn't enough cholesterol in the entire Amazon basin to clog up a single artery. (Then again, it occurred to me later, maybe they don't actually sell it, and that's why it's still on the shelves.) Unlike in the U.S., where stocks can be reliably and quickly replenished, here the transport system is sluggish and communication difficult. Many times since then I have gone to this same drugstore/warehouse and found the shelves filled with odd items like drops for "cerebral circulation" (don't ask me where or how these drops are administered to achieve their stated purpose) but vacant of useful antibiotics or the worm medicine that I desperately needed.

On this first visit, however, in addition to antibiotics, they also had an ample supply of disinfectants, worm pills, cough syrup, and the like. I spent a little over thirteen million intis (at that time, worth about $240) and collected a whole carton of medicines, along with iodine, cotton swabs, hydrogen peroxide, and so forth. When the proprietor, Eliseo, wrote up the receipt at the counter, he asked where we were going with all this medicine. Pam explained that we were stocking a clinic to treat the people who live near Yanamono Island. Eliseo then wrote *Clínica Yanamono* on the receipt, thus christening my off-the-wall venture.

Now the clinic would be more-or-less well equipped with the necessary medicines—and it had a name! We went off to celebrate the new enterprise.

# CHAPTER FOUR

# Jungle Medicine

As colorful as the story would be, no feather-bedecked shaman ever came to dance in front of me in an effort to chase away the blonde demon. The truth is that people appeared to be so desperate for medical help that they had been seeking medicines from Pam, who is a science teacher by training. They had been bringing their sick babies to her and requesting remedies for diarrhea, for skin problems, for wounds, and for a wide variety of other ailments. There were no requests to see my medical credentials (not at first, and never from the people themselves, only eventually from the health officials) and not even any effort to learn my name. In fact, I am still known to most people only as *la doctora.*

Patients continued to bring in a regular stream of common complaints, most of which after a short period of time I could handle easily. Once in a while, however, I was called on to deal with a challenge that was far more complex. I learned the most, of course, from these emergency situations.

Much of what I learned early on was that in jungle medicine "clean" was almost as good as "sterile," and "clean" was usually the

most I could hope for. Conditions in the rain forest are quite different from those that prevail in U.S. clinics and hospitals. When treating wounds in the field, sterile conditions are almost impossible.
When I packed my suitcases for Peru, I knew I was leaving the
world I was used to, and I thought I was coming prepared with
suitably scaled-down expectations. However, the reality was even
less than I had primed myself to expect.

When I set up shop here in the small room with thatched roof,
unwashable floor, and kerosene lamp, I wondered if I could actually
accomplish anything "medical" in this setting. But I was certainly
committed to trying. I aspired to make all the health-related procedures in my clinic as clean as I possibly could. However, I soon
learned that despite the less-than-perfect conditions, most people
healed quite well.

Here are a few cases in point:

A man approached Pam and me one morning to tell us his
wife had been in labor for over twenty-four hours. When we arrived
at their house, she was squatting in a corner over a none-too-clean
towel. A rod had been lashed diagonally across the corner of the
room on an upward slant, and she clung to this when her contractions came. The towel on the floor was soaked with the liquid of her
just-broken waters.

She looked tired of the whole thing. When her husband stood
behind her in the customary position, to do his part by reaching around
and pressing down on her swollen belly, she pushed his hands away
irritably. Finally, however, with Pam translating (I still needed Pam's
help, especially in emergencies) we got her to lie down. The woman
did not want to do so because the people here prefer squatting for
childbirth—which is fine for the woman but difficult for the doctor.

I rummaged in my bag, found a more or less sterile glove, and
examined the woman. I was able to locate the baby's head. I could
thus assure the waiting multitudes that the time was close and that
all we had to do was sit around and wait. Whether she was annoyed

by the intrusion or merely restless, I don't know, but the woman stood up again, paced a bit, and left the room. Within a few minutes, Pam, who had followed her, poked her head in the doorway and said, "Come quickly—she's doing it out here!"

She had resumed her squatting position back in the kitchen area, over a different scrap of discarded clothing. Suddenly she moaned, developed a look of intense concentration, and bore down hard. Her husband quickly took his place behind her; half-standing, half-crouching, he again wrapped his arms under hers, and put his hands on top of hers, and together they pushed hard on the top of the swollen uterus. The baby squirted out, slid gracefully onto its back and almost immediately began emitting angry cries.

The husband stood up, and the attendant women moved in and took charge of the infant. The mother leaned forward, panting a little but relieved and looking quietly satisfied. She reached down and tenderly wiped a little at her new daughter with a corner of the rag on which the child lay squalling vigorously.

Then, with another contraction, a gush of blood splatted through the slats of the floor onto the dirt below, and the placenta followed. I was curious as to just when the ritual would demand the cutting of the cord, but everything was left intact as the placenta was wrapped in one clean rag, and baby in another, and a third rag was given to the mother to tuck between her legs. The new arrival was carried, cord, placenta, and all, back to the walled room.

I remember this episode well because it introduced me to this area's less than ideal conditions of cleanliness and because it produced a goddaughter for Pam and me jointly. Just as important, perhaps, it also offered me a little reassurance that despite my strange foreign ideas about the preferred position for delivery, people accepted me anyway. This was confirmed on the way out, when Pam overheard one of the girls commenting on how the *doctora* had said that the baby would come, and the baby had promptly done so. My standing in the community was up a notch.

Another day, I was told that someone had cut himself with a machete and the cut wouldn't stop bleeding. Apply pressure, I advised. That had already been done, came the response. So I packed up a small set of instruments and suture material, and took my seat in the dugout canoe sent to fetch me. I found a boy of ten or so whimpering, moaning, and bleeding, his foot resting on a pile of blood-soaked rags while a friend held pressure on the wound.

It really was a mess. The cut itself wasn't too bad, maybe an inch and a half in length, just behind the ankle bone. But the child had managed to slash his posterior tibial artery, and every time the pressure was released, the wound spurted enthusiastically. There was at least a unit of blood (about a pint) on the rags, and who knew how much more on the path from the field where he had been working.

I started in on some serious cleaning. This meant lying on the floor next to the injured boy, along with the blood-soaked rags on which they had placed him. Chickens, as well as curious children and a dog or two, skittered through the house as the blood dripped down between the slats in the *pona* (palm fiber) floor. I asked for some boiled water (I was still pretty new here, or I would have known better), hoping thereby to obtain at least a semisterile cleansing solution. There was no boiled water, but a fire was started and a pot placed to boil. Meanwhile I said I'd settle for the regular water—straight from the stream we had just crossed.

The problem with arterial bleeding is always that it comes too fast to permit examination of the wound. Cut a vein and you can lose a lot of blood, but usually it comes out slowly enough that the source can be located by letting up pressure gradually and watching closely to see where the flow is coming from. With an artery, however, lighten the pressure and the whole wound is instantaneously awash. The best you can hope for is to spot the little pulsating spring and note where the blood is pumping out. There is only a fraction of a second in which to accomplish that before the pool is again too deep to identify the artery's exact location. This wound was pumping like a fire truck.

After six or eight tries, each separated from the next attempt by a good deal of sponging with my ever-diminishing supply of gauze, I could finally make out the severed vessel. It was two or three millimeters in diameter, not large, but since it was an artery, it was certainly capable of producing a brisk flow of blood. Once I could locate and identify it, it wasn't difficult to loop a suture around it and close off the flow from the wound. But I had hardly paid attention to the suture thread dragging across the floor and over the gore-laden rags—so much for sterile technique in this case. Also, there wasn't enough gauze or any larger sterile pieces of cloth left to make a sterile field, and that was that, so I simply proceeded, caring for the wound as best as I could.

I had one long, clean gauze bandage left, so I wrapped his foot like a mummy, cautioned him (and his mother) about the necessity of keeping it dry, made as tight a pressure dressing as I could, and instructed him to come back in five days and allow me to take out the sutures. Considering the lack of clean bandages, I left worrying about the risk of infection. However, when he returned, the wound had healed nicely.

On yet another occasion, I was whisked away to a house where I was told, "A baby has a splinter in his finger, and he can't urinate." At least that's what I thought the grandmother said. Remember my Spanish was still very shaky. When I dutifully examined the new-born boy, my splinter-in-the-finger interpretation began to seem doubtful. He appeared well. I pulled off his little socks, and there were no splinters there, nor in his tiny perfect hands.

Finally, I looked at the one part of the problem I was sure I had heard correctly—"can't urinate"—and there was my answer. The child's foreskin had no visible opening. The still air under the mosquito net suddenly got warmer. There is a saying in medicine: see one, do one, teach one; we docs are expected to learn quickly. Still, I kept thinking how nice it would have been to have at least seen one first.

Thank heaven I had packed a scalpel blade along with the instruments I had brought to extract a splinter (ha!). Conditions weren't ideal, but if this family could have gone to Iquitos, they would have done so already. I apologized to the tiny thing, swabbed his organ with iodine, injected a little lidocaine, and set to work. Thankfully, I had dropped a fine-pointed iris scissors into my field kit. I carefully snipped away a circlet of skin, revealing a tiny but perfectly formed male organ. (In the U.S., newborn circumcision is usually done with a little machine, not by hand.)

Then I swabbed away the blood, gave instructions for daily cleansing, left a few doses of antibiotics, and reassured the audience of family and friends that he'd be OK. They were still concerned because he had not immediately peed when the tip of his penis appeared. I explained that when the body is not taking in liquid, it conserves what it has. He needed to drink. The poor thing hadn't been fed since birth, and that was the real reason why he had not urinated. When I offered him my finger, he quit squalling and sucked hungrily, so I instructed the new mother to do what mothers always do, and packed up.

And so it went, in one palm-thatched house after another, as I did what I could, and my "practice" developed.

The biggest advances in modern medicine are not the dramatic, high-technology procedures like heart transplants, nor the fancy machines like CAT scanners, but the measures that address the spread of infectious diseases. Sterile conditions, hand washing, antibiotics—these are the measures that have affected the largest number of people and "saved" the largest number of lives.

But it seems to me that we may have reached a point, at least in the U.S. and other places in the forefront of modern medicine, where we have gone somewhat overboard. We have perhaps become excessive (or obsessive) in our collective desire to stamp out every last bacterium. I don't mean to say that there are no arenas in which that is necessary. Certainly, if we are going to perform organ transplants, or joint replacements, the highest possible levels of sterility must be maintained.

On the other hand, seeing how medicine is practiced in an environment lacking the tremendous advantages of any modern U.S. medical facility and seeing the overall outcomes (although I admit I use quite a few more antibiotics prophylactically here than I ever did in the U.S.), I am inclined to conclude that for most run-of-the-mill medical procedures—including the suturing of cuts and even the occasional cesarean section—clean is often very nearly as good as sterile.

Early on in my work here I lost my first patient.

The day had been busy. A woman with a tumor on the roof of her mouth came for a biopsy (actually on the prescribed day, a near-miracle given not only the lack of telephone or other readily available communication, but also the fact that she had to walk three-and-a-half hours through the forest from the Napo River to get here), a man came with a splinter in his finger, babies came in with diarrhea and ear infections—I was busy all morning. One of the patients was a fifteen-year-old boy, healthy the day before, with the onset that morning of nausea, vomiting, and diarrhea. I examined him and couldn't find much. He had no fever, his ears and nose and mouth were normal, his lungs were clear, his abdomen was benign (as we say in medicalese), there were a few mildly swollen lymph nodes at the back of his neck, and nothing else. I shrugged—not much to worry about here—pronounced viral gastroenteritis ("stomach flu"), and prescribed worm medicine and fluids. I reassured him and his mom, and they left.

In the afternoon, however, mother and son were back. I listened again to his lungs, heard wheezing everywhere, and knew we had trouble. But he was still moving air well, still had no fever, and he had no history of anything that sounded like asthma. I explained that sometimes people will have their first attack of asthma in conjunction with a bronchitis or even a viral illness, and gave him antibiotics and theophylline.

At dark, just before dinner, his father came, saying the boy was worse, and could hardly breathe at all. He wanted to know if he could give his son a shot, and held out two ampules of medicine that he had been told were "good for bronchitis." These were prettily colored, highly scented liquids, the snake oil of Peru. I answered as gently as I could that he could administer them if he wanted, but that they wouldn't cure his son. I gave him prednisone and albuterol syrup—more medicine for asthma—to take back to the house, but went to dinner with a furrowed brow. People can die of bad asthma, and I had no nebulizer (to administer medicine in the form of a mist), no oxygen, and certainly no ventilator (breathing machine). Should any of those become necessary, the boy was doomed. I didn't like the way this was shaping up.

At about one in the morning, the night watchman woke me. I struggled into clothes, grabbed my little flashlight, and hurried down the hall. The father was waiting in the anteroom outside the clinic. Juan Luís, his son, lay on the bench, swathed from head to toe in a sheet. To avoid moving him, I brought out the stethoscope and kerosene lamp and examined him where he lay. He still had no fever, but fever would have been more encouraging than his damp, cool skin, which already had nearly the waxy feel of a dead body. He was completely alert and aware, unfortunately, and when I put the stethoscope against his chest I found that his lungs were nothing but a mass of rales and crackles. He no longer sounded wheezy like asthma, he sounded like he had a raging pneumonia. Or it could have been pulmonary edema, fluid backing up in the lungs due to a failing heart (an x-ray would certainly have been welcome), but he had no other signs of heart failure, and no heart murmur either now or earlier in the day.

A normal respiratory rate is twelve to twenty times a minute; that is how fast we usually breathe. He was breathing eighty times each minute and struggling desperately for each breath.

I tried, unsuccessfully, to get an injection of ceftriaxone, a sort of superantibiotic, into a vein. Then I decided to move him after all into the bed in the clinic and give him some fluid intravenously— partly to fill his pitifully empty veins, partly to reassure his father. It took a couple of tries but I finally got the liquid flowing in and gave him the antibiotic. But it did him no good. He cooperated as well as he could, but he was obviously horribly uncomfortable and unable to breathe in any position. He kept saying, "*No puedo resistir*" ("I can't take any more") and kept breathing nearly as rapidly as his heart was beating.

While the fluid dripped into his vein, I took his father out to the *sala*. I didn't want to say, "Look, your son is dying and I can't do a thing about it," but we both were aware of the way it stood. I said that he was "*bien grave*" (really sick) and that I thought that there was nothing more I could do. I had already given him all the drugs I could think of that were available to me. Oxygen, more antibiotics, aminophylline, steroids, beta agonists by inhaler or nebulizer, ultimately a ventilator, were all things I should have used, and would have if I had them. But I didn't.

All this, of course, is assuming it actually was asthma. If this was a case of congestive heart failure after all, then my intravenous fluid wasn't helping him, and a diuretic would have. On the other hand, if it was indeed asthma, the diuretic would have been detrimental, and the fluid necessary. There are simple tools that would have helped me to differentiate more certainly between those two possibilities, but those weren't available, either.

There was nothing else I could offer except to stand around and be useless; nothing more to do except watch as he struggled for breath until he couldn't struggle anymore. His father seemed to be entertaining thoughts of trying to get up to Indiana, and I encouraged that. It probably wouldn't make the slightest difference to the patient himself, but the family might be comforted by the fuss that would be made over him there, and at least there would be various medical persons, instead of just one, hanging around and looking grim. I warned the man, though, that I didn't think Juan Luís's chances were good, period.

They departed, the father carrying the bundle, almost as large as he was, that was his eldest son. I went back to my room and huddled, thinking about futility. In the morning, when I walked past Raúl, one of the waiters at the lodge, he reported, "The kid died," and it turned out that he had done so in his house, in the predawn hours.

In the U.S. when a patient dies, rarely does the physician call on the bereaved family. We have already moved on to the next patient, and unless you know the family well it may seem like an intrusion on their grief; besides, the family may wonder whether the doctor is there out of a sense of guilt or failure. So usually our care ends at the deathbed and stops short of the graveside.

Here, I knew even less about customs and expectations. I did not know if my presence at the home might seem like an admission of something, but these people were more than my patients, they were community.

So I crossed the stream and went to their house—well, actually to their neighbor's house, their own being little more than a dirt-floored hut. The neighbors had offered the use of their *sala* for the *velorio* (vigil), which is the important preburial rite here. I wanted most of all to give the boy's mother my sympathy.

When I arrived, there were thirty or forty people sitting on the benches around the open room: men on the left, women and children on the right, a spontaneous division. No one particularly seemed glad to see me, but then it was hardly a glad occasion, and no one, at least, looked as though they held me to blame for this death. Juan Luís lay on a table jutting out into the room from the back wall, covered with a sheet from his feet to his shoulders. Candles burned on the four corners of the table.

From behind the wall rose a wailing song, or a singing wail, one voice raised in a half-sung, half-chanted expression of loss and grief. I asked if it was permissible for me to join her. Reassurance was given that there would be no problem with this; I passed through the opening that served as doorway, to find the bereaved mother leaning against the wall opposite the point where her son lay in the other room and wearing the clothes she had worn when she had come to the clinic the day before. She held a towel against her face as she moaned her infinitely sad song. I think she made it up as she went; it didn't seem to rhyme or follow a pattern, but it was none-theless compelling and melodic: "Oh, my son is gone . . . never will I see him again . . . never be with him again . . . never hear him returning to me again . . . he has left . . ." and on and on, probably for hours, in the language that Hemingway called the most roman-tic and beautiful.

I was a little surprised to find her completely alone, but maybe she chose it that way. I stood for a moment at her side, but she was unaware of me. Then I reached over, touched her shoulder, and slid my arm around her, and she let me pull her close. After a few moments she looked up (she didn't come much past my shoul-der), and I was relieved to find no chastisement in her eyes, only grief, which I shared. She put her head on my shoulder and cried, never stopping her song, and I held her and cried a little too. Then I left her to her solitary mourning. She nodded slightly at me before replacing the towel over her face and leaning tiredly again up against the wall.

I followed the sound of the hammer and saw back to the kitchen, where the coffin was being constructed, delivered the Valium I had brought to help the bereaved mother sleep, and went back out.

As I left the house, one of the mourners attached herself to me, following me back to the clinic for an office visit, or *consulta*. She made me feel that I hadn't completely lost the people's confidence as a result of this failure, and that seemed like something of value. It was good for me to be near someone as well, since I felt the ache of grief and the powerlessness of medical failure.

# CHAPTER FIVE

# Indiana

All this time, I was practicing medicine essentially without a license. Officially my medical degree from the University of Wisconsin and my Wisconsin license carried no more weight here than a Peruvian medical degree and membership in the Peruvian Medical College would have carried in the U.S. It therefore seemed prudent that I ingratiate myself with the medical system of the region.

To this end I began to schedule some time at the clinic in Indiana. Indiana, halfway between my clinic at Yanamono and the city of Iquitos, is about twenty-five miles away, or an hour and a half by boat. Indiana is also the location of the Explorama Inn, another of the network of ecotourism facilities operated by Peter Jenson. According to a monument in the town square, Indiana was founded in the late 1940s by a French Canadian Catholic mission-ary, who envisioned it as a "model settlement for all of Amazonia." Apparently, the man from whom the site was purchased had actu-ally attended school in Indianapolis, Indiana, so that was the name chosen for the new community.

Its two or three thousand inhabitants make Indiana the only town of any size in the whole area surrounding Iquitos. The founding fathers built a church, a school, housing for both priests and nuns, and a medical center. Over the years, as support from home parishes in North America dropped off, the mission's size dwindled. By the time I arrived on the scene, although the church was still active, the two-story, block-long priests' home had only a few residents, and the medical center had been turned over to the Peruvian government. One or two nuns still served the *posta* (rural medical center) alongside the government-paid medical staff.

Services at the *posta* were overseen by a police nurse. There had not been a doctor there for several years. The nurse's presence constituted a recent upgrade in service, although the corps of aides, more or less equivalent to LPNs, had shown themselves to be quite capable, having weathered many years in which there had simply been no higher authority. I found Gaby, the nurse, to be a fount of information, and I devoured her advice on common illnesses and their customary treatments. Furthermore, she was a gracious and pleasant person as well as a competent practitioner. Although the lines of authority did not appear to be very clearly laid out, Gaby was aided by the *auxiliares* and by Madre Carmela. The latter, a nun who counted some eighteen years of experience at the *posta,* later confided to me that she had never had any sort of nursing or other medical training. The *posta* had been promised both a general practitioner and an obstetrician, but no one had said when they might be expected to arrive; the Peruvian government had virtually no resources, financial or otherwise. The administrator, Jaime, held the keys to everything needed by Gaby, Madre Carmela, and the *auxiliares,* and had some omnipresent but never clearly defined authority over all the doings of the *posta.*

The *posta,* known optimistically as a hospital, was the only real medical facility within hundreds of square miles. It served thousands of people, but led a precarious existence with minimal help from the church, a little support from the regional government, and precious little else.

When Pam and I first went to Indiana, we had arrived at the airy, balcony-surrounded house that was home to the few remaining nuns. Madre Carmela appeared to have no reservations about my serving at the *posta* as long as Gaby didn't object. I would eat and sleep at the inn, Explorama's nearby facility, and walk each day to Indiana. The local people, on the whole, cautiously welcomed me. As Gaby was about to complete her year's service and return to Iquitos, the idea of a doctor on site must have been appealing. On the other hand, apart from my obvious incompetence in Spanish, they knew nothing about me, not even whether I was a real doctor as I claimed. They were realistic enough to recognize that it was a little unusual for a physician in the U.S. to abandon a practice there in order to come to the jungle.

For my part, I was mildly terrified at the prospect of being so isolated, once Pam left. No one would be available to translate for me as they did in Yanamono, and to date I had been speaking Spanish for less than two months. Further, it was not clear to me how much medicine was available, how one would obtain more, or how effective the support services were. There appeared to be no way to move a patient deemed too ill for the facility. In short, I was facing all the disadvantages of Yanamono, but on unknown turf and with the specter of governmental involvement lurking somewhere in the background.

But I did want to begin to familiarize myself with the local practice of medicine and, in turn, let the medical authorities in the region begin to get to know me via the river-connected grapevine. So after our first visit I packed a few days' worth of clothes, bid a temporary good-bye to my room and my crude clinic at Yanamono, and went, all by myself, to Indiana. I felt like a kid going off to school for the first time, and I think Pam felt like a mom watching her child set out on her own.

Arriving at the *posta*, I found two of the *auxiliares* and Jaime, the administrator, all looking unoccupied in the reception area. In clumsy Spanish, I introduced myself and told them of my conversation with Madre Carmela, and they agreed that I could hang out for a while. Terese, one of the *auxiliares,* took me on a tour of the facility.

The *posta,* judging from its style, must have been constructed in the late fifties or early sixties. It is a one-story building replete with standard medical areas: pharmacy, procedure room, doctor's office, small laboratory, and surgery room. I also noted two rooms for patients, a room used for new mothers, a closet/cleaning supplies room, a linen room, a kitchen, and a screened-in area built across the narrow end of the building. This would become the space for cholera cots when that malady made its appearance a couple of years later, but it was unused when I first arrived there.

Despite the nice building, however, the *posta* was clearly designed for a medical system with much greater resources. For example, the linen room and pharmacy were locked, and the keys were jealously guarded by Jaime. Once inside the linen room, I saw no more than a small stack of sheets, a wash basin, and an unused treadle-operated sewing machine. Continuing on, I found the pharmacy heavy on injectable potassium, lidocaine, and chloramphenicol, a potent but somewhat dangerous antibiotic rarely used now in the U.S. There were very few useful medicines. Two or three pairs of exam gloves, a few sets of IV tubing, and a half dozen liters of IV fluid sat on the partly filled shelves. It appeared that I would have to either take my chances on the small general stores in the town that carried pharmaceutical supplies or bring medicines myself from Yanamono.

The furnishings in the patient rooms were sparse: no curtains, no pillows on the beds, no tanks of oxygen. Running water, collected from a rooftop rain-gutter system, flowed into the sinks in each room. But the plumbing did not reach the toilets; flushing required filling a basin from the sink and pouring it into the commode. Electricity ran only from dusk to midnight, when the town's generator was operating. Consequently, the autoclave used to sterilize distilled water, gloves, suture material, and metal instruments ran only in the evenings. There was no refrigerator and no x-ray machine. The very competent laboratory technician had no reagents with which to work, much less machines to test cholesterol, liver enzyme levels, or electrolytes, and no facilities to do blood cultures. He did show me a microscope, a hand-operated centrifuge, and a twenty-year-old text on medicine—in English. I hid my dismay at the difference between these sparse resources and what I had hoped to find in the "small government hospital" at Indiana.

After all, I reminded myself, the *posta* was a decent facility, despite the water stains and tropical mold climbing the walls, and it had a corps of experienced and very competent workers.

Several people were hospitalized at the time. We stopped by the bedside of a young man who was being treated for arthritis. I looked at his allegedly arthritic knee and was surprised to find it neither red nor swollen nor painful nor crunchy on movement. Puzzled, I asked him if it hurt, to which he admitted that no, it really didn't. By definition, arthritis is an affliction of the joints, and his seemed normal. Trying to pin down the problem, I learned that he couldn't walk. But why not? He had been walking until recently. He had had no injuries. The muscle mass in the legs had not deteriorated. So, I asked him to try standing . . . and he crumpled to the floor, or would have if Terese and I had not been holding him. I performed simple muscle testing—now push, now squeeze—and found that his hands were also very weak. I checked for deep tendon reflexes with my hand, since I did not have a reflex hammer (I could see I was going to have to bring my own instrument bag, as well). No response.

This was looking like Guillain-Barré syndrome, a malfunction of the nerves that control the muscles, that is, a type of paralysis. It usually follows a viral illness, though no one really knows how or why. It doesn't affect the nerves of sensation, so feeling remains intact, as was true with this young man. It is self-limited and usually passes without causing serious problems other than a few weeks of inconvenience and the very frightening sensation of losing control over your body. Once in a while, it advances to the point where it affects the muscles of breathing, but as I tried to explain the disease, I didn't mention that. If it went that far, the patient would die, since the *posta* did not possess a breathing machine. Why bring it up? Besides, he had been there for several weeks, so the illness had probably already progressed as far as it was going to.

I did suggest that they quit giving him intravenous antiinflammatory medicines and steroids, which would only cost his family money they couldn't afford.

The other patients were a couple of people with abscesses, both receiving ampicillin, and a lady with vomiting and intermittent abdominal pain that I couldn't account for. All in all, I was pleased to find three out of four patients for whom I could at least do a little something.

We then spent an hour or two folding pieces of gauze cloth into the small squares used to clean wounds, dab at blood, swab the skin with alcohol, and perform other such mundane and common medical tasks. In the U.S., these gauze pads come prefolded and sterilely packaged from some unseen factory, but here we cut them from cloth and fold them by hand when there isn't other work for which we are needed. The cutting and folding allowed us to chat amiably if awkwardly. The two aides, Consuela and Terese, despite only two years of nurse's aide training, were quite competent. Soon we had haltingly established our respective ages, marital statuses, and number of children. They were surprised to hear that I had no children, as it is virtually unheard of here for a healthy woman past the age of thirty not to have children. They both, despite their Catholic upbringing, were using birth control—tubal ligation for one, birth control pills for the other. They seemed pleased to have a doctor around and wanted to know how long I'd be working there and how often I would come back.

It had been a pleasant afternoon, and only a little scary. We agreed that I'd return in the morning, when Gaby would be present. Except for my apprehension at having to contradict her diagnoses and treatment plans (the patients with abscesses really needed more than ampicillin, and the young man with "arthritis" certainly did not need antiinflammatories), I was looking forward to it.

Then I set off to walk home. The hospital is at the edge of town, so I passed the plaza, houses, taverns, housefront stores, and a boat being constructed in a long open shed near the river. It reminded me of Noah's ark. Of course, here the river rises to flood stage every year, and so would soon enough come to pick up this boat.

At the end of this stretch, the road took an uphill turn and headed off through what amounted to the suburbs of Indiana. Here the cement sidewalk ran for a block or two before giving way to a corduroy path—logs laid crosswise in the mud—and then, finally, to trodden dirt. A broad grassy space was bordered by houses and was alive with soccer games, people out for evening walks, and small groups socializing as they returned from work in the fields. I ran into a young man who worked at the inn, out promenading with his wife and baby, who smiled at me in cheerful recognition and indicated that I was indeed on the right path. I also picked up a couple of temporary companions: two young women who laughed at how briskly I was walking and pointed out how much more slowly the Peruvians stroll. After realizing that they did mean to accompany me and that they were scrambling to keep up, I slowed my pace and we went on together. When we came to the last of the houses, they waved good-bye and turned off the path. All along my route, everyone politely murmured *buenas tardes* (good afternoon), and I murmured the same back, trying without much success to get the same trill in the *r*s that everyone else rolled off without effort.

The dirt path wound uphill and then down again, through fields of banana and *yuca* crops (manioc, not the rosette-shaped yucca plants of the North American Southwest), and crossed gullies and small streams bridged by narrow poles a few inches in diameter. In a couple of places the path rose to a panoramic view of the river. Houses became more and more sparse until there was a long uninhabited stretch with forest looming on the hills rising beyond the cultivated fields. Then I arrived at the inn, where I spent a pleasant, relaxed evening.

In the morning I trekked back to Indiana, again attracting much interest along the way, but already beginning to feel like a familiar figure. Word must have spread, because a man accosted me on the path and asked if I would stop to see a patient. I agreed somewhat reluctantly to do so, as I was still very much aware of my unorthodox and not clearly defined professional status. I tried to explain to him that, although I was a physician in the U.S., I was really no more than a visitor here. But one of the problems with learning a new language is that one can not always convey exactly what one intends to say—and people tend to hear what they want to hear, anyway. I was led into his home up a gangplank, which I interpreted as a sign of a poorer household, since most other homes had front stairs made of a notched log. The patient was a young but very tired-looking woman with a two-day history of fever and bloody dysentery. Probably a bacterial infection, I thought. I explained the precaution of boiling river water before drinking and promised to bring antibiotics on my way back at noontime, assuming there were some available at the *posta*. Before I left, they insisted that I take a couple of delicious bananas and a papaya.

Arriving at the hospital, I was warmly welcomed and offered a cup of sweet milk with a little coffee in it. The first patient was a woman in her eighth month of pregnancy (with her ninth child). Consuela asked if I would care to examine her. She seemed fine on exam, at least as far as I, a specialist in internal medicine, could tell. The baby's head was down but not yet engaged in the pelvis, meaning that, thank heaven, she wasn't yet in labor. I asked for an obstetric stethoscope to listen for the fetal heart, half expecting to receive the portable Doppler ultrasound machine I had used a few times for that purpose in Wisconsin. Instead, I was handed a little wooden trumpet about eight inches long with a hollowed-out center. To my pleasant surprise, using this old-fashioned instrument I was actually able to hear the tiny heartbeat.

After seeing a few more patients I walked home for lunch, stopping on the way to deliver the promised antibiotics to the grateful woman I had visited earlier. At dusk I returned to the *posta* carrying enough chicken, rice, bread, and fried plantains for three people, kindly whipped up for me by the obliging cook at the inn.

Back at the *posta*, I tended to a few more patients and settled in for the night. The room that had been prepared for me was a chamber whose largest dimension was its ten-foot-high ceiling. An iron bedstead was fitted with one sheet and a pillow, no blanket. Someone had thoughtfully draped a sheet over the window that looked onto the waiting room. At that point I could not have said exactly why I was there, but it somehow seemed that I needed to be "on call" to establish myself as a part of this system—at least for one night.

I passed a quiet night from midnight on, once the town's electricity was turned off, bringing a halt to the radio supplying the music for the fiesta next door. The next day I left Indiana and returned to Yanamono.

A routine soon developed: I would spend half the week at the Yanamono Lodge, where I had come to feel at home in the fledgling Clínica Yanamono, and the other half of the week at Indiana, where I continued to feel like a boarder, however welcome.

Four times a day at Indiana I hiked the four kilometers between the clinic, where I worked, and the inn, where I ate and slept. When I left the inn in the morning, the dew hanging on the leaves was sucked off by the sun before I reached the outskirts of town. Before I even left the inn, perspiration was beading up on my forehead. If it had rained in the night there would be some mud on the jungle path, but the clay was well packed and edged with coarse grass. In Indiana proper, it was another story altogether. The grass was worn away by the many feet passing daily, and the heavy red clay stuck in great clumps to my shoes. These masses grew larger with every step and, with amazing tenacity, never fell off spontaneously. This same path provided little shelter from the sweltering afternoon sun during my walks to and from lunch.

On the last lap of the day, however, the walk always seemed more charming. The sun would be low and setting around the time I reached the inn, so there was some shade for relief and the air was cooler. By that time, of course, I had already finished a day's work and was headed for a cool shower, fresh clothes, and a good dinner. The inhabitants of the village, also finished with work for the day, often grinned and called to me as I passed by. The smoke from the cooking fires drifted its homey scent across the path. Sometimes a harvest of rice was spread out on the sidewalk to dry, or bumper crops of fish were filleted open and lay drying in the sun on racks of split palm. The smoky smell of the drying meat mingled with the other flavors in the air. All along the trail myriad children played, drawing hopscotch blocks on the sidewalk with pieces of charcoal stolen from the cooking fires, setting up miniature soccer games with tiny balls, or simply sitting or standing and watching.

Past the town and into the forest, the shadows lengthened. When I came up over the rises, great piles of clouds were often lit up by the sun setting ahead of me. And by the time I reached the inn, the sky would be soft shades of pink and violet and orange, silhouetting the tall, frothy palms. As I contemplated the end of the day it was easy to think of this place as a tropical paradise and to reflect that I was, after all, right where I needed to be.

Working in Indiana, however, was not my ultimate goal and was often frustrating. I was far from a radio, telephone, fax (ha!), or any other method of communication. Leaving the Indiana clinic doctor-less during the night made me feel derelict in my duty, but living there would have been awkward at best, considering the accommodations. The physician's house adjacent to the *posta* was now home to a number of the *posta's* employees, and it would have seemed ungracious of me to displace everyone. Besides, the lack of separation between work and rest was one of the many factors that made it so difficult to convince a Peruvian doctor to stay in such places.

The scarcity of patients also bothered me. I was becoming known in the region around Yanamono, and more and more people were coming to my small clinic there. Yet, despite the *posta's* vastly larger and better-staffed facility, few people came, in part because they didn't expect a doctor to be there. Why paddle your canoe for three or four hours if the doctor will probably not be there anyway?

The real problem was not one of demand, but of supply. If I settled at Indiana permanently, patients would eventually come. But there were virtually no medicines in the pharmacy aside from those I brought. Theoretically, all that should have been necessary was a request to Iquitos for the needed supplies, but in the usual diversion of practice from theory, repeated requests had yielded nothing. The *posta* was essentially government-operated, despite the nominal contributions of the mission, and at the time the president's policies and personal expenditures had all but cleaned out the government treasury. I could not personally take on the responsibility of stocking a facility that, if it ever got up and running, could easily see five hundred patients a month.

So, I concluded that my medical practice would need to stay centered downstream in Yanamono.

Working at Indiana was a good learning experience, and served as the entree I had wanted into the local health care system. It was also an introduction to the state of affairs, generally, of that system. Visitors here sometimes ask what I do about patients too ill for me to handle, expecting that I will respond that I somehow evacuate them to Indiana or to Iquitos. But, problems of transport aside, conditions in the regional clinics and hospitals (the only ones even potentially affordable for my patients) are marginal at best.

So, having gotten my foot in the door of the official system, I retreated to Yanamono to try to improve my unsanctioned version of rural health care.

I also contacted my medical partners back in Wisconsin and told them that I would not be returning: I wanted to extend my three-month leave of absence by a year. Now the bridges were all burned. It looked like I was here to stay.

Life on the Amazon

# CHAPTER SIX

# Life Along the Stream

Stepping off the plane in Iquitos, you can have no doubt that you have arrived in the tropics. Warm, heavy, unmistakably tropical air engulfs you, thickening as you descend the ramp steps. If it's night when you land, there may be a moon wavering in the hazy sky. If it's daytime, the sun will be beating down and the heat will be billowing off the tarmac.

You almost inevitably arrive by stepping out of a plane. You can't come by rail; there are no tracks through the thousands of miles of surrounding forest. Nor can you come by car or bus or taxi; there are no roads longer than three miles—the one that goes out to the airport. You could get here by boat, but that would mean that you had come 2,300 miles up the Amazon, from its mouth in Brazil, unless you were hardy enough to have followed the tricky paths down the eastern slopes of the Andes and then taken a series of boats via the Ucayali or Marañon or Huallaga River. In that case, if you hadn't perished along the way (and you wouldn't be the first to have done so), you could arrive by boat from upstream.

Mostly, nowadays, anyone from outside the immediate area comes in by plane. There are daily flights to and from Lima (and from there to and from the rest of the world), and one each week from Miami direct to Iquitos. The latter is pretty much reliable now, rarely more than one or two hours late.

They've modernized the airport, but they haven't gotten around to working out a system for passing people through customs, so international flights are chaos. A line forms, everyone goes by the Immigrations personnel, who stamp the passports, then everyone is left milling around in a large, open room, with no clue as to what comes next. The luggage usually takes about half an eternity to begin dribbling in, and since the tour operators aren't allowed to enter this area, the arriving tourists have to figure out on their own that they must locate and claim their bags, then queue up again for customs inspection, after which they drag their stuff out the front door into the humid night, not knowing that the tour agencies who are expecting them are all crowded around the exit doors waiting to claim them.

From the airport, it's a half-hour ride into the main part of the city, in either a *motokar* (a half-motorcycle, half-rickshaw affair that is the main taxi substitute in Iquitos) or a bus (with windows that drop inside the wall of the bus when it's not raining and a windshield that props up out of the way to let the balmy air sweep through). From the air, there are no lights to be seen as you approach the city, despite its considerable size, but as you drive in from the airport, you notice that the forest has been cleared from the surrounding hills and that shacks, huts, and hovels have replaced the trees for a mile or two on either side of the highway.

The food market offers river turtle and caiman meat (sadly, both endangered now) and fish ranging from small to the two- or three-meter-long *paiche*, including various kinds of catfish and piranha (delicious when fried). There are also plenty of sweet and hot peppers, cucumbers, eggs, chickens, tomatoes, entrails of various animals, and a marvelous array of fruits and vegetables never seen in U.S. grocery stores. Individual stands sell everything else you might need— plastic housewares, shoes, sandals, soap, clothing, and sewing supplies. Other stands offer a varied menu of finger foods—for example, balls of rice packed around a scrap of seasoned chicken, wrapped in a *bijau* leaf and boiled. These are called *juanis,* after San Juan, on whose feast day they were originally served. Other ready-made lunches include *tacacho,* balls of mashed-up roasted plantain seasoned with salt and pork cracklings; *tamales,* small oblong packets of ground corn and peanuts wrapped around a shred or two of meat and boiled in a *bijau* leaf; dishes of rice with fish or chicken; fried plantains; and *empanadas,* small fried turnovers of boiled and mashed *yuca* formed around a little chicken and a few vegetables. In the midst of all this, *ambulantes* (walking vendors) roam through the crowd, hawking brooms, balloons, mothballs, mirrors, whatever can be carried in their hands or over their shoulders. The scene is energetic, picturesque—and noisy.

Since most people have no refrigerators or pantries (nor the money to keep them stocked), every day is market day, and crowds mill around shopping from about 6:00 A.M. until 6:00 P.M., that is daylight hours, every day of the week, though it's usually a bit less crowded on Sundays and holidays.

Leaving the city behind, Explorama uses thatch-roofed boats called *pamacaris* to transport its guests to the lodge. These are just like the river taxis used by the local folks . . . with several exceptions. Tourists have the benefit of cushions on the seats, a restroom in back (a sort of outhouse built behind the motor, which can be an adventure to get to), a thermos chest full of soda and beer, a good motor and a reliable source of gasoline, a nonstop ride, and a distinct absence of chickens, cows, baskets of produce, and other domestic wildlife and market fodder crowding the floor of the boat. The typical river taxis may take four to six hours to travel the fifty miles downriver to Yanamono Stream, but in Explorama's boats the trip is about two-and-a-half hours. It would be faster by car, if there were roads—although if there were roads, they'd be Peruvian, not

North American—so on second thought it might take a couple of days, especially if it was raining.

The river is broad and usually almost glassily smooth, even though a powerful current clips along at four or five miles per hour. I saw a newspaper article once in which the author referred to the "lazy, slow-moving Amazon" and wondered which Amazon he'd been visiting. Traffic is constant, ranging from small dugout canoes to the ocean traffickers, from the double-decker launches, slung with hammocks and crowded with people, chickens, and other wildlife, that ply the river to Colombia and Brazil, to the open boats, powered by outboard motors, that are the main transport system for the local economy. The motors on these boats are small but tremendously reliable, with long sweeping tails culminating in tiny propellers. The boats aren't speedy but are excellent for navigating the maze of shallow waterways that run into the main river.

Life around here is, of course, governed by the river, which is absolutely and inevitably a part of everyone's daily life. The sheer volume of water that it carries is almost incomprehensible, and for one who lives in the U.S., the changes it goes through annually are likewise difficult to truly understand. Tourists who visit here in August, when the river is down and we cannot bring boats on the stream all the way in to Explorama and must instead park on the Amazon and walk in, have a hard time picturing how it must be when the water is deep enough to bring the big boats directly to the dining hall. Those who come at high water, on the other hand, find it impossible to imagine a time when the stream cannot be entered. The change in water level is routinely twenty to thirty feet and can be as much as forty feet, and although the magnitude of change varies from year to year, the cycle occurs annually without exception.

The Iquitos area is what is called an "ever-wet tropical rain forest." That means that we do not have distinct "dry" and "wet" seasons. It rains, on average, about two days out of every three, for a total of about 120 inches of rain a year. There may be spells for a couple of weeks without rain, or several weeks in a row when the sun never seems to make an appearance, but these may occur at any time. Furthermore, although the torrential rains of one night may raise the stream by several feet the following day, that water quickly runs off; the following day the stream returns to whatever its baseline was. The main river is affected less by the rain that falls on this area (which is fairly consistent year round) than by what happens hundreds of miles away in the Andes, where thousands of small streams converge to form dozens of small rivers that in turn combine to become a half-dozen large rivers and finally merge into the two great ones whose confluence defines the beginning of the Amazon proper. It is at the meeting of the Río Ucayali with the Río Marañon, not far upstream from Iquitos, that the Amazon River proper begins. (In Brazil, the Amazon is said to start at the conjunction of the Río Negro with our Amazon, but we know better.)

Peru is south of the Equator, although just barely. Summer in the mountains is, therefore, November through February. The glaciers melt, rains fall, and the runoff collects in the many tributaries that eventually empty into the Amazon. In the Iquitos region the water begins to rise usually in October, and generally by November the boats can once again enter Yanamono Stream. The water continues to rise until its peak in mid-May, after which it falls abruptly as the glaciers freeze up again and the mountain precipitation changes from rain to snow. Usually by late June, the stream is again too low to admit the boats. It drops to a trickle by July and stays that way until September or October, when the cycle begins again.

This dramatic cycle necessitates certain adjustments in living arrangements. Homes are built on stilts or pilings, four or five feet off the ground, and even at that, those on lower-lying land may have to be abandoned in years of especially high floods. (A few homes, notably in the Belén sector of Iquitos and some of the "gas stations" along the river, are built on rafts and simply spend their entire lives on water—rising and falling with the seasonal "tide" of the river.) Steps from the homes down to the river are cut into the banks with a machete; each year the water washes away last year's steps and new ones must be chopped out when the waters fall again. At the clinic, this creates a bit of a problem: how do you carry a sick, weak person up a slippery bank that may be as much as thirty feet high, with a steep incline? If we build steps, either they are washed away or their footings are rearranged by the rising waters. On the other hand, no steps at all is a real nuisance, especially when the water is dropping and the steep bank is oozy mud. Our solution was provided by the *huatchimanes* (Spanglish word for "watchmen," although they really do far more than that), who devised a set of movable staircases each six or eight feet in length. They put the sections out or take them away according to the needs dictated by the river. The steps sometimes sit at peculiar angles, since they are built at one angle and the bank's angle may change from time to time. But overall, they work pretty well.

Fields are planted with the flooding in mind—as the water falls, rice, beans, watermelon, and other crops are sowed on the banks. By the time the water rises, it is time to harvest. (Clearly, any unusual delay in the dropping of the water or unusually early rising may imperil the crops. Fields on slightly higher land that is only sometimes flooded have the advantage of periodic renewal of their soil, but risk crop loss in the years that the floods inundate those fields.)

Navigation on the river is also affected. It is easy to tell whether the river is rising or falling, even without looking at the banks: if it is coming up, it is full of floating debris. Whatever was dropped along the banks the last time the water fell is picked up and moved on out. There is, of course, no way to control what falls into the water as the banks crumble, and it is not unusual to see an entire banana tree, fruit and all, lying lazily on its side as it is swept down the river. For the boatmen, it is a difficult and sometimes dangerous prospect to navigate as the water is rising. Not only is there plenty of the riverine grass floating in clumps and little islands, excellent for fouling a propeller, but entire trees, some of them rain-forest giants, are occasionally seen as well. Even worse are the trees not seen . . . there are sometimes deadheads, floating beneath the surface of the muddy water without a trace showing above. Hit one of those and your propeller simply shears the pin that connects it to the motor, leaving you stranded in the water—not an uncommon occurrence.

Then again, there are certain advantages to the water's rapid rises. The clumps of floating grass and water lettuce and water hyacinth are not all that gets washed out of the blackwater lakes as the river comes up. Sometimes fish can be seen jumping in silvery flashes; this indicates a *mijano* (school of fish) swept out from some inland lake now connected to the river. Word is passed from one neighbor to the next, and pretty soon everyone is down by the river throwing their cast nets to capture dinner and, perhaps, also enough fish to smoke or preserve by salting.

The extent of the area covered by the flooding is astonishing. The lodge is located about fifteen-minutes' walk inland from the edge of the Amazon. In years of very high water, everything from the dining room all the way out to the river is inundated. This amounts to hundreds of square miles of seasonally flooded land in the area between the lodge and Iquitos alone.

When the water falls again, it has left behind a layer of mud up to six inches deep that goes through several stages before finally drying to hardpan. First there is the water-on-top stage, with standing water covering the silty muck. Walking in this is tricky not only because of the obstacles (and occasionally animals, like the stingrays that frequent shallow waters and carry a terrible stinger that leaves a wound festering for weeks), but also because the mud is as slick as potter's clay, and when your foot smooshes through it trying to find footing on the solid earth below, the bottom layer is slipperier than glare ice.

Next comes the stage when the puddles are gone, but a lot of moisture is still mixed in with the silt. At this point, the mud has the color and texture of supersmooth chocolate frosting, and it is not too hard to wade through except for the continuing slickness.

The third stage is the most difficult. When enough of the water has evaporated to congeal the mess a bit, but it is still nowhere near solid, then every step you take is a sinking, sucking one, with the mud attempting to pull off your boots, if you wear boots, or the little buried sticks and so forth waiting to ambush your soles, if you wear feet. It all makes for terrible walking for the first few weeks after the river goes down, especially if there happens to be a rainy spell in those weeks.

Along the Amazon shore, the vista is green and more green, although much of the vegetation downstream from Iquitos is second growth. The original rain forest has long ago been cut and replaced with sugarcane, bananas, and *yuca*, which are the staple foods here. Small houses, made of palm slats, roofed with palm thatch, and raised on stilts to avoid the annual flooding, line the edge of the river. The farther downriver you go, however, the more scattered the houses become. From the river the landscape looks fairly well populated. But everyone lives either right on the river edge or very close to it. No one wants to live more than a few meters from the source of their drinking water and cooking water, their bathtub and laundry, their playground and parking lot. So if you want isolation, just head inland away from the river and you'll get away from people in no time. You will, in fact, escape all traces of civilization, for better or worse.

In addition to watching for floating debris, riverboat captains need to keep an eye out for unexpected sandbars, which occasionally crop up even close to the deepest channels, for fishermen and their nets (watch for floating pieces of old sandals or empty plastic jugs or oil barrels, any of which may be used as markers or floats for the nets), and for people in dugout canoes, whose upper edges are perilously close to the water and which can be swamped by even a relatively small wake.

In this area the water itself is a soft muddy brown, colored by the clay that the river collects from the banks and the fields upstream. But let this water sit for a day or two in a jar and it becomes crystal clear, with a thin layer of mud at the bottom.

The sky always holds clouds. With thousands of square miles of rain forest, the transpiration from all the billions of leaves from all the millions of trees creates a continuous supply of puffy cumulus clouds. Almost daily, these dissolve into rain showers. And when the equatorial sun shines, it beats down fiercely. Even Florida-tanned skin will burn in half an hour—on a cloudy day.

Yanamono Stream, on which the Explorama Lodge is located, flows into the Amazon from the west (the left if you are going downstream, which, confusingly, is north). Yanamono Island is ten or twelve miles long and splits the river into two channels. The channel on our side is smaller but still a good half mile across. In June or July, the water gets low enough so that it's impossible to enter the stream, even in a dugout canoe. Most of the year, however, the boats can enter the stream, so I can float straight in to the steps leading up to my *casa* (house).

The Yagua village is on the left of the stream as you enter it from the Amazon. The village consists of a settlement of thirty or forty small houses and a population of 150 to 200, plus a grade school and a small secondary school. The primary school is one room with clapboard siding, cement floor, and tin roof, built by Explorama as a gift to the community; the secondary school is a one-room, thatched-roof, dirt-floored building, about twenty by forty feet, with a few benches inside.

A typical *casa* sits on a bare patch of dirt extending ten or twenty feet in every direction. The nakedness of the "yard" has nothing to do with aesthetics—it has to do with survival. If the vegetation is allowed to approach the house, the termites, which I am told constitute the largest biomass in the forest and which are a constant threat to any wood product, come with it. Worse, "snake in the grass" is not just a figure of speech here. Everyone knows someone, often a family member, who has died of snakebite, besides several other friends or relatives who were bitten but survived. It's neither wise nor healthy to invite them into your home. So the area surrounding the house is conscientiously kept clear. A few homes have gardens of herbs and/or medicinal plants, though in general the fields *(chacras)* in which the *yuca* and plantains are cultivated are farther inland, on land too far from the river to be suitable for housing.

Each house is built on stilts four to five feet off the ground, in order to be out of the way of the yearly flood waters. In some years my house is accessible only by canoe for a month or two. During those times, I can hear fish jumping in the water at night, beneath my bedroom floor.

Floors are usually made of *pona* slats, which are durable, somewhat flexible, and spaced slightly apart leaving openings in the floor—a perfect arrangement for the babies, who rarely sport diapers. Anything spilled or dribbled simply goes through to the ground below. The size of the house varies according to the size of the family who lives there, and to some extent also according to the family's prosperity. The better-off families have larger houses, occasionally even with plank floors. A typical *casa* housing a typical family— father, mother, four to seven children, an in-law or two, and sometimes a few extra kids or other relatives—will be about fifteen or twenty feet wide, and twenty to thirty feet long.

The *casa* is generally divided into two rooms. In front is an open living-playing-eating-socializing area called the *sala*. This open porch-like room is likely to have a railing around its periphery, and sometimes also a couple of benches for sitting, as well as a hammock. The hammock is the favored spot for general relaxation and serves as an excellent crib. Interior decoration is sometimes provided in the form of the glittery remnants of the last fiesta held there, be it from a birthday or Easter or Christmas. Sometimes a colorful calendar or magazine clippings or outdated newspapers decorate the walls. Some families have acquired a tinted photograph or painted portrait of one of the adults, looking solemn, vague, and Peruvian Gothic, which will be hung in a highly visible place of honor.

The room in back is usually smaller and is separated from the front of the house by a wall or a screen. This wall may be constructed of planks or more *pona* or maybe a palisade of wild cane. The room is usually enclosed, though it may be left open in back. Neither this room nor the one in front has a ceiling; above the rafters of peeled slender logs the thatch roof looms in the shadows. The back room is used for sleeping. Few families have a wooden bedstead, and if they do, it is very rare to see a mattress on it. More commonly the family simply sleeps on the floor. In the daytime, the mosquito nets are slung up over the rafters; at dusk they are unwound and lowered over the beds, which consist of a pile of clothes placed on the hard floor to soften it. The mosquito net hangs tentlike over the bedding and voila! sleeping quarters. Children sleep with their parents until the age of three or four or five, and often they're not the only ones sharing the grown-ups' bed. I saw a woman not long ago whose infant had a skin disease. I wanted to treat everyone who was in contact with the baby, so I asked her who slept in the bed with the child. Her answer: herself, her husband, and her father-in-law.

Given the lack of privacy, I sometimes wonder how there can be as many children as there are here. I think, though, that when it comes to intimate activity, the keywords are quick and quiet.

Another mosquito net or two or three in the same room will house any remaining children, plus whatever in-laws, guests, or other strays are staying in the house that night. It is not out of the ordinary for someone you've never laid eyes on to show up on your step, explaining that he is your wife's second cousin's neighbor-in-law, and that he and his wife and children would like to camp out with you for a while. Such requests are rarely refused.

Whatever possessions the family owns will be arrayed along the walls of the back room or stashed in the rafters above. These will include a few clothes, perhaps a fishing net, maybe a shotgun or—in the more traditional homes—a blowgun, a basket or two, and whatever odds and ends the family has accumulated. There is never very much. There may be a half dozen articles of clothing hung along the walls, and perhaps a backpack for trips to the city. These items, along with the utensils used for cooking and eating, make up the poorer family's entire stock of possessions. People need little else to live here, and in any case don't have money for luxuries.

The kitchen is either a corner of the *sala* or, in the nicer homes, a platform separated from the rest of the house, to avoid the danger of fire. The stove consists of a patch of dirt and ashes formed into a rectangle on the floor, topped with several slender logs arranged Lincoln-log style, with a metal grill laid across the top. Sometimes a platform has been built at one side of the hearth to serve as a work area. It is not unusual to find the lady of the household squatting on top of her stove in the morning, stirring the pot of river water, fish, and plantains or *yuca* that will be the family's food for the day. Most families have three or four large pots and a collection of plastic plates, soup bowls, and cups, along with a few spoons and a kitchen knife. The machete is put to use in the kitchen as well as everywhere else. Most families eat at a table fashioned by the man of the house, with a bench alongside, but it is not unusual to find a home without these niceties.

Needless to say, these houses do not have indoor plumbing. A few families and a few communities have dug latrines, but often exercising one's bodily functions is simply a matter of finding a secluded spot in the forest, nothing more.

Nightfall, naturally, signals the end of the day. Unless there is enough money to buy a flashlight, or a little kerosene to fill the small lamps made of discarded coffee cans with wicks of rags, the houses are dark. Daylight means time to wake up and go to the local "grocery store"—the family's small field or the muddy but fish-filled river.

In the *ribereño* communities, the houses are scattered along the riverbanks, sometimes for a mile or two. Each is home to one family, although, of course, that family is probably extended—sometimes very extended. In the Yagua village across the stream from my house, many of the old ways of living are still observed. The entire village was once housed in a single communal house, called a *maloka,* with a rounded roof that extended to the ground. In the village today, separate houses remain clustered more or less together, with the schoolhouse at the center. The soccer field is the large rough open area located at one side of the school.

Every village, no matter how small, has its soccer field. When you spot a collection of two or three houses at the river's edge, you can be sure there will invariably be an open space between them with goalposts of crude sticks marking the boundaries. In the city, kids play *futbol* (soccer) in the streets, using clumps of grass to indicate the goal area and dodging traffic as they kick and run.

Somewhere in the village, one house will have an oval shield on the front with the governmental emblem painted on it. This is the home of the local governor. Near it will be a small, open-front shed; this is the jail used for men who have become overly rowdy at the fiestas, overtly beaten their wives, or failed to show up for one of the community work projects such as cleaning or painting the school or clearing paths through the village.

In the larger villages, there will be a house or two that sells soap, canned milk, cigarettes, sugarcane rum, and other supplies, but no real grocery store—and certainly no gas station or church or bank.

This is a poor area, and the towns are basically places to live and work the fields—no theaters, golf courses, or bowling alleys here. Hundreds of thousands of people live in communities such as these, scattered along the waterways of the lowland jungle. The people by and large appear content. These days, there is some movement into the city by those looking for better education for their children or better work for themselves; yet there is also movement from the city to the rural areas by those who have found no work in the city.

The Indians mostly wear clothes now, the old languages are fast disappearing, and the makers of blowguns are becoming ever fewer. Nonetheless, life along the river flows along pretty much as it has for the last few generations, and although the city and its ways are not far away on the map, they are still distant from the day-to-day patterns of life here.

CHAPTER SEVEN

# Life Outside the Clinic

The first few years I lived here, whenever I felt down, tired, discouraged, isolated, lonely, or just plain ready for a change, I would sneak off and ramble down the lodge's trails that wander through gorgeous scenery. The Bushmaster Trail goes out from the back of the lodge and heads off into the stretch of jungle between the Amazon and the Napo Rivers. Ten minutes into the Bushmaster, one is out of earshot of anything whatsoever that is man-made. Not even the rumble of the largest and loudest of the river barges penetrates this part of the forest. Local folks say that a three-hour walk from the Bushmaster leads to the Napo River. One visiting scientist, however, ambitiously set out to walk that path one day. He took a local guide, since going alone through uninhabited forest along a nearly invisible trail is a certain way to become hopelessly lost. He returned after a very long day without ever having reached the Napo.

Merely walking out onto the Bushmaster for a while is enough to unwind my wrangled nerves. The peacefulness of that green cathedral emanates from every tree and liana and is only underscored by the forest sounds. My personal favorite is the call of the toucan, a single, high, piercing, melodic note that carries for long distances through the canopy.

The Lake Trail leads to a blackwater lake after passing through primary rain forest. It floods almost every year but is home to immense trees. There is one kapok tree that must be more than twenty feet in circumference. Nearby stands the giant ficus with a skirt of buttress roots from which we swung on vines during my first visit to the forest. The lake itself, typical of oxbow lakes common to this part of the Amazon basin, is a remnant of what was once a bend in the riverbed. The water constantly reworks the riverbanks, cutting away the outside edges of curves and depositing soil on the inside edges. Every so often, a hairpin turn becomes so narrow at its base that it is simply cut through and left behind. This rerouting of the river forms oxbow, or blackwater, lakes. Their water truly is black and, unlike the Amazon's, is as clear as strong tea. Their dark coloration is due to the leaching of tannins from the vegetation rotting in their depths, and their clarity is due to the lack of current. No soil crumbles into the water as it does in the main river. Wondrous creatures live in the blackwater lakes—electric eels, caimans, and many kinds of fish who swim amongst gigantic *Victoria amazonia* water lilies. The bizarre hoatzin birds, thought to be unchanged from prehistoric times, live at the edges. Their young tumble from the nest into the water when threatened and are born with claws on their wings so that they can climb back up. Mystery always seems to surround these isolated depths of still water.

In some years, it is possible to take a dugout canoe along the Lake Trail. This is fairly simple: just follow the part of the water that doesn't have trees emerging from it. However, the trail poses special obstacles when flooded. Branches, leaves, and vines that are normally overhead are now at face level and must be either ducked under or swept aside. Ducking is a nuisance, but sweeping the branches aside invites fire ants, large spiders, thorns, angry wasps, and other undesirable passengers to drop into the canoe.

The occasional fallen tree also necessitates a sometimes complicated and tricky detour.

The water trail also looks very different from the dry land path. In most places the trail is wide enough, and the brush on both sides thick enough, to distinguish what is trail and what is not. In some places, however, the undergrowth thins out and a watery plaza opens up. Here, trees ranging from saplings to monsters loom up out of the murky water, and the route is not readily visible. The landscape, so familiar as a trail during the dry season, seems foreign in the canoe. It is easy to become lost. I proceed very cautiously.

During one paddle into this area, I came across a snake swimming in rapid S curves. He was only a meter or two ahead of me, headed in a direction that would cross my path. When he finally noticed my approach, he looked to be as startled as I was—his eyebrows flew up, and he immediately dove, disappearing beneath the water's surface.

As you emerge from the forest trail into the lake, the sudden opening offers a startling view. It is at once quiet, idyllic, and mystical. Most of the time, the lake is covered with a thick mat of grasses and small trees. When the rainy season raises the water to a certain level, a reunion occurs with the main river and all the vegetation is carried on out into the river. Then the lake looks like a secret hidden pond, with glossy black water, deep blue sky overhead, and dense emerald forest all around.

Not a bad way to spend an afternoon, if you have one.

For me, the problem is that nowadays I rarely have free afternoons. When I first opened my "practice," patients arrived in combinations of ones and twos—sometimes as many as a half-dozen per day, but occasionally none at all. If no one was waiting when I finished breakfast in the morning, I simply took off and explored the area. As business picked up I began to adhere to set clinic hours. Now I often spend my free time at the house, waiting for the next call from the clinic.

One good friend, who has known me for many years, wondered aloud how an energetic person like me could endure the laid-back, serene, and tranquil life of the rain forest. "Hah!" I replied.

My world here is physically smaller than the world I inhabited in Wisconsin, where my house and my office were separated by a twelve-mile drive. Here at Explorama the lodge, the clinic, the spaces in between, and the surrounding rainforest are all within easy walking or canoeing distance of each other.

The lodge sits on the banks of Yanamono Stream, a tributary of the Amazon River except during flood season, when the Amazon itself flows through it. The lodge is a collection of buildings similar to most local native construction. The lodge's four guest houses comfortably hold 120 tourists. One house is available for guides. A dining hall also accommodates employees in a back extension. Most employees live in the city and work here in two-week to three-week periods before returning to their homes in the city for a few days off. The Bar Tahuampa also serves as gift shop, social club, and music hall. The joyous music is supplied by one or two official musicians and an ever-changing backup band of guides, boat drivers, barmen, and room boys. They play one or two guitars and a rich variety of percussive instruments: a pair of maracas, spoons, a *cajón* (a small box that the percussionist sits on and beats with his hands), and occasionally a large metal flashlight whose circumferential ridges create a washboard sound when the performer runs his fingernails over them.

Kerosene lanterns light the bar, dining room, tourist quarters, kitchen, and my room. Small smudge pots are also set along the paths between the buildings.

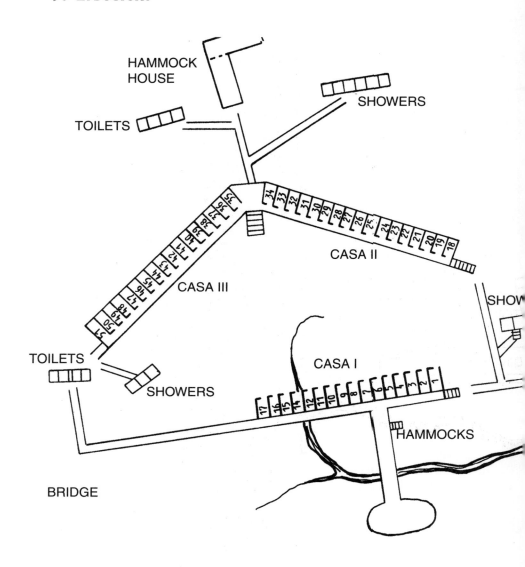

**EXPLORAMA LODGE**

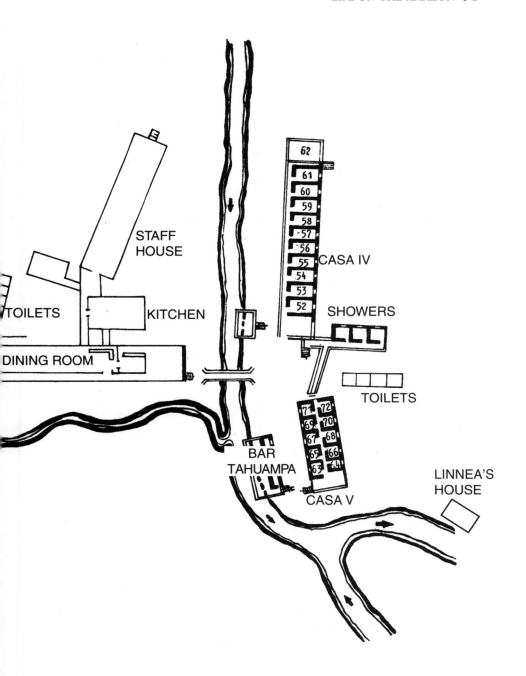

The lodge has running water in the showers—gravity feed from a tank high on a hill—but no indoor plumbing. Sometimes the pump that brings water from the stream to the storage tank runs amok. That poses a significant problem. Lodge staff then enter into urgent radio consultation with the Iquitos pump mechanic, who brings his heavy bag of tools and spare parts from the city in a motorboat. Direct communication with the office in Iquitos, some fifty miles away, is only by unreliable shortwave radio. At times, attempts at conversation are drowned out by static or the transmissions of extraneous conversations in other parts of the jungle. The post office box that I claim as my address actually belongs to Explorama and is located in Iquitos. We have neither postal delivery nor phone service in the rain forest.

My quarters have no cooking facilities, but that's OK with me. The kitchen behind the dining room receives regular supplies of fresh fruit, vegetables, meat, rice, canned milk, and other perishable food by boat from Iquitos, as there is no market or grocery store anywhere in this area. Explorama's cooks work miracles on a kerosene-fired stove, although the contraption makes me nervous. Its top measures two by six feet, with three industrial-size burners and a poorly working oven. Pressurized kerosene is held in a metal tank charged by a piston, which must be pumped vigorously prior to lighting the stove and occasionally thereafter. In the predawn coolness, the cook can often be seen pumping away, with the pilot light flame soaring up to two or three feet in height. In the wavering light of the flame, surrounded by the shadows of the darkened kitchen, the cook's face glows with perspiration. Highlighted by vivid light contrasting with deep shadow, he looks like one of hell's minions busy at work.

I eat my meals with the tourists when there are any; otherwise I eat in the kitchen with the employees. On one of the latter occasions, upon entering the kitchen, I found a whole small animal lying paws-up in a roasting pan. It had sharp teeth, small front paws, and heavy hindquarters, and resembled a miniature tyrannosaurus. "What is it?" I asked, to which they replied, "*Está carne del monte, Doctora*"—jungle meat.

It was delicious.

The sounds of a city do not penetrate here. Both the sounds and the animate life of the forest, however, make their presence continually known. Termites, for instance, are a constant threat. They must be fought vigilantly. A sighting of their crumbly, above-ground tunnels, built in straggling trails up the pilings beneath the house or winding along the underside of the stairway, is a call to immediate action. They travel from nests in trees, down the trunk, along the ground, up into a house, and aim for the roof. They are nearly impossible to evict once in residence in the palm thatch, and the damage they wreak is significant. The roof on a friend's house actually collapsed while he was away, its rafters weakened by the termites ensconced there. Here most houses last for only a few years before they must be rebuilt. People find it difficult to believe that a house can actually endure for a century, as they do in North America.

I use the local approach to termites: douse all of their trails with a little squirt bottle of kerosene. Later, after the kerosene has done its work, I scrape off the debris with a machete, so that new termites cannot move undetected into the old tunnels. Even better is to use insecticide. When I spray the little devils, I get rid of the ones there today while also providing some protection against future incursions—at least for the short-range future. Before too long, however, the entire process starts over again.

The *cucarachas* (cockroaches) are also everywhere. Their leavings, dirty little brown spots on scraps of paper and little holes chewed in clothing, are annoying. I detest them. I have, however, learned a strategy that sometimes foils them. They apparently don't like mothballs any more than moths do, so I regularly sprinkle the small white spheres in drawers and among clothing. I even put them in my typewriter, since it is a favorite hiding place of theirs. Strange as it is to have a typewriter that smells like naphthalene, the odor is preferable to the alternative—roaches jumping out whenever I start to type a letter.

The plant life must be dealt with as well, lest it overcome house and yard. Quick-growing weeds that surround the house are vehicles for opportunistic termites and dangerous snakes, and must be regularly scraped away. Algae thrive on the plastic screens around the open upper half of my walls. Removing the green-gray patches is equivalent to washing windows in Wisconsin. But I only washed windows once a year, at most. Here my screens must be scrubbed inside and out every two to four months, depending on how much rain and how little sun we've had. If unchecked, the jungle will take over with unbelievable speed. Here, I'm afraid, "jungle rot" is not a literary exaggeration.

On the other hand, I seldom shovel snow. Then again, my roof requires constant maintenance and upkeep. The entire house is built around a frame of skinned poles. At the level of the rafters, the poles terminate and the rafters are laid across them and lashed in place with durable, flexible vines, called *tamshi*. From the horizontal poles, others are raised at an angle from either side, to meet at the ridge of the roof. A ridgepole runs horizontally across the top, connecting and stabilizing the other supports, all of which are tied together with the same *tamshi* vines. A framework is then constructed on these supports, over which lengths of thatch are lashed into place.

The thatch itself is a fairly interesting bit of construction. It is built around a thin, square pole about eight feet in length, called a *crisneja*. A species of palm found along the Napo River is knotted at close intervals along the *crisneja*, using the stem of the leaf to tie it onto the pole and leaving the overlapping leaves hanging down.

Seventy or eighty leaves are woven in this manner onto each *crisneja*. Each *crisneja* sells for about fifty cents, which makes me glad that I do not earn my living making them. Hundreds of *crisnejas* are needed to make a single roof. The roof's life span depends on how closely the thatch is laid. If made well, the roof will last four or five years before the rains have beaten off enough pieces of the thatched leaves to allow significant leaks.

Patching can extend the roof's life for another year or two, so I periodically require this service. A small repair crew that worked on my roof one day consisted of two agile young men supervised by Octavio, who looks exactly like Santa Claus without a beard. Without any sort of ladder, the young men put one foot on the edge of the window and hoisted themselves into the rafters. From there, they scrambled up to the next level of rafters and arranged a couple of long planks into a platform on which a chair was placed. I half expected one of them to do a handstand on the chair and juggle plates with his feet.

Instead, Octavio handed up a *crisneja,* which was swung up to the makeshift scaffolding. One of the men then shinnied up one of the angled roof-support poles. He clamped his knees around the pole, wedged his back between it and the roof, poked the *crisneja* between two others, maneuvered it into place, and lashed it to the roof supports. For the most part, Octavio coached and scolded from the floor, "No, no, the other way! Do it right, now!"—although he wasn't above clambering into the rafters himself every now and then, despite his fifty-odd years. I became dizzy just watching them. They walked lightly across the round, thin rafters as if they were on firm ground, and I was filled with admiration.

There is no ceiling between my living quarters and the roofing thatch. Small debris tends to sift down—dust loosened by little lizards scurrying through, occasional fragments of the dry thatch leaves, frog droppings, and every once in a while a discarded snake skin. One day I found a silky white sac, about the size of a tennis ball, collapsed on the floor in the midst of fifteen or twenty baby tarantulas. Each was cute and fuzzy, only about one-half-inch long, but already looking like a miniature of its grown-up self, complete with pink toes.

I share the house with Otoronga, a miscellaneous mixed-breed cat whom I adopted after her mother had abandoned her in a muddy ditch at two weeks of age. Her name means "jaguar" in the Yagua tongue—a fitting name because, like all cats, she believes that she is a mighty predator.

Her propensity for hunting is sometimes a nuisance. She doesn't present me with her prizes, thank heaven, but does enjoy using the round plastic laundry tub as a small arena for the torture and killing of small lizards, frogs, and so forth. Every now and then, a strange smell will hover around the room, prompting me to track down and remove the leftover meal that has been abandoned once she has eaten all she wants of it. When the water is high, she is also an accomplished fisherwoman.

Early one spring the stone man came. The little raft from which he sells his inventory of stones was spotted floating down from upriver, and word spread from house to house along the river's edge. When he arrived everyone went out to welcome him. The *huatchimanes* wanted to buy a stone for the clinic.

The stone man's arrival causes such a stir because there is no rock in this part of the Amazon—none at all. Thus, in order to sharpen your machete (the tool employed daily for cultivating the crops, chopping up the dinner, building and repairing the house, and myriad other uses), you must buy a stone. This fellow was the vendor. By midday, the little docking site in front of the steps by my house was so full of dugout canoes it looked like a mall parking lot in mid-December. Everyone came across from the village to check out the stone man's wares.

The stones he carries are gray, smooth, flattened lumps of rock that look like big wads of dough and range in size from about two fists to two gallons. The sugarcane mill located on the corner where Yanamono Stream runs into the Amazon has a venerable old one that is closer to three or four gallons in size, green on the sides with moss accumulated over the years, and flattened on the top, where countless machete blades have been rubbed over it. The stones are sold by the kilogram. The clinic bought one about a gallon in size for S/10.00 (ten soles, now worth about $3.50).

The fellow's name was Luís. I met him because he came into the clinic with a fever and a headache, thinking he had malaria. When I looked into his ears, however, I discovered that both ears were infected. I explained this to him and assured him that not all fevers are caused by malaria.

I then asked him about his work. He said that he built his raft in Yurimaguas, up on the Huallaga River, where he lives. This is a great distance away, virtually in the foothills of the Andes. From there, he floated down to the Río Marañon and from there to the Amazon. He will go downriver as far as Pevas, a hundred miles or more downstream from here, stopping all along the way to sell his cargo. At Pevas, he will abandon the raft and take a launch back upriver. The whole trip takes him a month and a half, and he completes it about twice a year. He invited me to come and see his raft, so after work, I took him up on the offer.

When I arrived, several kids were standing around looking on, and occasionally adults came by to make purchases. The raft was about ten by twenty feet, with a deck raised about a foot above the base and a simple tent in the center. The tent's roof was made of blue plastic covered by palm thatch, and the centerpole was tall enough so that the man could sit up in the center, if he bent down a little. His bedding and a few—very few—odds and ends were spread on the deck inside. The back end of the tent was closed, and the front was open; he sat cross-legged in the doorway of his small domain, awaiting his customers. The open hearth he used for cooking was built onto one front corner of the raft, and a jumble of pots and pans were tumbled together along the outside edge of the tent. A small cage on another corner of the deck held chickens that he buys or takes in trade and that probably constitute the major part of his diet for his journey. His stones were piled on the open deck on both sides of the tent. He left Yurimaguas with about five hundred stones and was down to about two hundred by the time he reached Yanamono. He looked relaxed and comfortable sitting in the front of his tiny tent, and I wished him a safe and successful journey.

Although I am clearly not a native here, local people have shown me great kindness and acceptance. I am invited to graduations and birthday parties, where no one seems to notice that I am the only blonde, the only really light-skinned person, and the only woman bumping my head on the rafters.

One year, Olga and Juvencio invited me to share Christmas with them. On the afternoon of Christmas Eve, Juvencio looked jittery. He confided that his problems had begun in the early morning, when the rooster he intended to butcher for the main course had escaped into the jungle. This was the first time he and Olga were to host a major holiday gathering, and he wanted it to be a success. He wondered aloud if the other chicken he had on hand would be enough to feed all the guests at the celebration. I cautiously asked how many invitees there were. "Fourteen," he said. I suggested that obtaining a second chicken might be a good idea.

By midafternoon, his spirits had improved. He had managed to acquire a rooster from a neighbor after promising to hand over the escapee once it was captured. I loaned him a dollar to buy sugar for preparing *chicha*, a drink made of corn meal boiled with sugar and left to ferment. I can't stand drinking it, but he and Olga love the stuff. Since they had no money for purchasing Christmas ornaments, we took a few balloons from the clinic and twisted them into parrots, dogs, and fish and hung them in the rafters, to the delight of the watching children. Olga requested that I bring a paper napkin with me when I came that night. It seemed to me like an odd request (only one?) but I didn't want to pry, so I just agreed.

Pouring rain had come down the previous night, leaving the path between our houses a mess. I slowly navigated my way to their house and offered the presents I'd brought: earrings for Olga, a Swiss army knife for Juvencio, chocolate for their three children. Only then did I remember that I had forgotten the napkin. Although the return trip to the lodge was icky and I still hadn't an inkling what they wanted with a single napkin, they had made a point of asking me to bring it. I went back to fetch the requested item. A few other people drifted in after an hour or two, and the *chicha* was passed around. When even more people arrived they started up the generator back in the kitchen, music spewed forth from the stereo, and dancing began.

At midnight, the traditional hour for Christmas dinner, Juvencio invited me into the kitchen. Their small table seated only eight people at a time, and there were actually about thirty people in the house, so I felt honored to be among the first round of guests to be served. On the table, plastic picnic plates bore a token piece of rooster (tougher than shoe leather, but wonderful flavor), a small scoop of stuffing, a hunk of boiled manioc, a piece of *panetón* (sweet bread sprinkled with raisins and other dried fruits, which here replaces Christmas cookies), and a plastic fork. Every guest also received a cup of hot chocolate, and at my place, I found the lone napkin I had brought from the lodge.

The opening of the champagne capped off the festivities. Champagne is readily available in Iquitos around the holiday season and goes for about a dollar a bottle. It is sticky and sweet and only slightly bubbly: probably, all in all, the worst champagne in the world. But it, too, is traditional.  Even though the bottle was shaken briskly before opening, the plastic cork fell limply into the hand of the man opening it. But the toasts offered were warm with good cheer, and the feeling of being at home among friends was unmistakable.

# CHAPTER EIGHT

# Red Tape

Some people who visit Peru are struck by the same impulse that felled me and want, somehow, to help. "What medicines, what supplies, can we send you?" they inquire. "You can't send anything," I reply. "You can only bring things when you return. Your friends who follow in your footsteps, impressed by your adventures here, can bring things when they come. But you cannot send things."

They want to know why. Will nothing arrive through the postal system? Well, that is part of it. Although recent improvements have been made, not everything that enters the labyrinthine passages of the Peruvian mail system emerges intact at the receiving end, if it emerges at all. But the real problem is the customs office.

I received word early one October that four boxes of medicines had arrived for me at the post office. The closest post office branch is in Iquitos—fifty miles away, or four hours by boat.

On my next trip to the city a couple of weeks later, I stopped in at the post office downtown. Yes, they had four boxes with my name on them. No, I could not have the boxes. *Aduana* (customs) must release them to me. The customs warehouse and offices, where incoming ships unload their cargoes, is in the Punchana district on the edge of town. I went to the port area and immediately spotted the man I needed to talk with. He did not appear to be otherwise occupied. At first, he responded to my request by informing me that they handled post office stuff only on Tuesday mornings, or more precisely, during two hours on Tuesday mornings. He explained that there was simply not enough manpower to do it every day, and certainly not enough manpower to do it right now. Then he seemed to think it over and asked if I had a vehicle. Upon hearing an affirmative, he said, "OK, let's go."

He balked again when he saw the little Honda 125 motorcycle that is my Iquitos transport. It appears that he was laid up for a year after one cycle accident and never rides the things anymore. I offered to hail a motorcar. He considered that option for a moment, then sighed and resignedly climbed on the back of my bike.

I drove with extra caution through the seemingly unregulated confusion that is traffic in Iquitos, and we discussed the awful state of drivers and driving in the city. He asked my name. After a few minutes, he remembered having read an article on my work at the clinic that had appeared in *Ojo*, a daily newspaper that is like a hybrid of a tabloid and a serious paper. Actually, I and my patients were in the centerfold, and I was dramatically dubbed "The Angel of the River People." *Ojo* always has a scantily clad female on the cover, but legitimate news stories, reports of political activities, sports, and comics are included inside. The issue with me in it had briefly made me famous, at least locally.

We stopped along the way to deliver some papers of his, which I suspected to be his real reason for coming along. He thanked me for the errand, and I thanked him for helping me.

At the post office, he unlocked the room where the boxes were sequestered. We took the cartons down from the shelves, dumped the entire contents out on a tabletop, and took inventory under the supervision of a post office representative. There was not as much medicine as four boxes had given me to hope. All of it was samples: small packets that drug representatives leave with doctors to influence us to use the latest in whatever they are peddling. In other words, there was a lot of packing and only a few pills in each package. But it was still a significant quantity of pharmaceuticals, and it certainly made an impressive pile on the post office table.

As we sorted through it all, the *aduana* man noted the inventory and replaced it in the box—or at least most of it. People seem to revel in an assortment of ailments, and everyone absolutely adores *remedios* (medicines). In a country where literally anything medical can be bought over the counter, without a prescription, self-treatment is rampant. In fact, pharmacists often recommend treatment, even if the patient is not present, and most pharmacies offer free injection of any drug they sell. The man found the antibiotics and iron pills most intriguing. The antifungal creams also had appeal, and each man kept a couple of the small tubes. Then he asked, "What's this with the picture of the kidneys on it?" "That is an antibiotic," I replied hesitantly. "Can I have some?" he asked. "I have a kidney stone." I explained that the medicine would help neither a kidney stone nor low back pain, only a urinary infection, but he still looked wistfully at the package each time that little drawing of the kidney came up.

The *aduana* man's mother consumed a great quantity of antacids, he explained, so he was thrilled with a couple small bottles of Mylanta, and positively beamed when I offered a few rolls of Tums as well. The post office fellow was sure he had high blood pressure. I asked how high. He responded, "Oh, it's OK now," so I asked what medicine he was taking for it. He answered, probably quite truthfully, "Oh, all kinds!" Not surprisingly, anything I identified as high-blood-pressure pills really attracted him. He was a bit let down to be told that he actually needed to have his blood pressure measured prior to initiating treatment, so I consoled him with some Tums.

Finally the three of us had sorted through the entire shipment and stuffed most of it back into the boxes. The boxes were then replaced on the shelf, and the *aduana* man let me drive him back to Punchana. He promised to fill out the necessary papers and have everything ready by the next morning.

I was hoping that there would be no customs duties to pay. After all, the donated medicines were only samples and were destined for the poverty-stricken people downriver. I was fairly sure that there should be none legally, but I was not at all positive. In any case, what is written in the books doesn't always govern what goes on at the docks. Still, the *aduana* man had professed admiration for the noble work I was doing and thanked me graciously for the medicines he had collected.

I dutifully showed up at *aduana* headquarters in Punchana the following day. I didn't see my friend of the day before, and was told I needed to talk to "*la señora*," a woman who was supposed to arrive soon but wasn't yet in. I settled onto a wooden bench and passed the time by writing in my journal. In this way I continued to pass time for "one minute more" until an hour and a half had gone by. Then, the *señora* arrived. Unfortunately, once she finished shuffling and tapping and leveling and generally organizing the papers in front of her, she wanted the equivalent of around $80.00 to turn the medicines loose. Although they would easily have been worth more than that if bought retail, I wasn't about to buy them retail. They would all be useful, but I wasn't immediately suffering for lack of any of them, and I hated to start a habit of paying ransom for such donations.

So I protested—gently, I hoped—and was soon escorted to another customs administrator. The office to which I was sent contained the head of the *aduana* enclave, who was absolutely unhelpful. He suggested that I apply to the regional government for an exemption, but could offer no more details. He could not give me a name, a title, an office, or even a department to whom I should appeal, and Iquitos is home to dozens of governmental agencies and bodies.

The man who had initially completed the inventory paper-work with me, to whom I had given the sample medicine, was a bit more helpful. He supplied me with the name of another customs official in a downtown office, across the street from the post office, and further mentioned a document that I should request: something called an "Exoneration of Customs Fees."

It was now close to noon. I hurried, since no one in any sort of government office around here works past the midday break. On my arrival downtown, the customs office there informed me that the gentleman I was seeking was out at the warehouse in Punchana, where I had just spent the morning. He would be in the office in the afternoon, they asserted.

I surrendered the round and returned downriver to my clinic.

Later that month, I found myself back in the city. The man I sought was not in the office on my first trip to the downtown customs office. He was also not in on my second visit, even though I sat for two hours in the anteroom, glancing up every time any-one approached the door. Finally, however, I managed to catch up with him. He politely invited me into his office, waved me into a seat, and expressed his boundless admiration for my work. He even presented a copy of the *Ojo* article tucked into a folder. However, in the  most congenial, most gracious, and most appreciative terms, he told me that he couldn't help me. I needed to speak with a gentleman who worked at—where else—the *aduana* office in Punchana.

I trekked back to Punchana, where I was in luck, sort of. When I arrived, the man I needed was actually present in his office and not otherwise occupied. He was also most supportive of my efforts, but his hands were tied by the law. He gave an "it's beyond me" shrug and said he could do nothing without a request from the president of the Regional Government of Loreto. I was directed to submit a request to said president, who would in his turn direct *aduana*, who would then be delighted to turn the boxes over to me, in full accordance with the law.

I retreated to Explorama's office, where the secretary obligingly typed up an official-sounding *pedido* (request) for the needed exoneration. When I took it to the building where I had been told the Regional Government was headquartered, I found out that the president actually worked elsewhere. I backtracked, located the building, was admitted through a wrought-iron gate by a military-looking guard, and sat down to wait in a reception office. The lady who finally came to attend me showed me upstairs, past another guard, where I sat down to wait again, this time in the office of the president himself. An elegant executive secretary glanced with lightly disguised contempt at my *pedido* and informed me that they could not possibly approve such a request for an individual. Well, I could understand that. They had no way of knowing if I were indeed practicing medicine in the jungle. After a bit of negotiating, she conceded that they probably could honor a request for exoneration if it was made by UTES, the agency responsible for health care in the rural areas. I never laid eyes on the president himself.

I traveled from there to the Hospitál Iquitos on the far side of town. The people in UTES, thankfully, knew me from previous contacts. When I explained my problem and offered to split the proceeds with them, they willingly typed up a *constancia*— essentially a certificate that pronounced me their representative in this matter.

Back at the office of the president, I was soundly rebuffed again. First, I made the doorkeeper angry by mistakenly handing her my original request. Her offended response was a Spanish version of "Why are you bringing me this old thing again?" Realizing my error, I offered her the new, improved *constancia* from my folder. She remained firmly unmollified. They did not want a *constancia*. They needed a *solicitud* (a petition, more formal than a mere *pedido*) and a separate letter stating the donor's name and address, plus a detailed list of the boxes' contents. She had already TOLD me that, she glowered. Actually, my limited grasp of Spanish was not sufficient to her instructions, but I had been too intimidated to request that she repeat everything.

I returned to UTES, where I found everyone at lunch across the street. I accepted their jovial invitation to join them, which was probably good public relations, but when we returned to the hospital, the typist was nowhere to be found.

I gave up for the day and found a room for the evening.

The next morning I reported once again to UTES. Again I waited, this time for a Señor Vargas. When he arrived, he gave the typist instructions. I peeked at the sheet as it unfurled from the typewriter. "Solicitud," it said at the top, followed by an approximate list of the medicines we were trying to ransom. Good. I trooped back across town again. I sailed past the gatekeeper and the guards, smiled at the helpful girl in the downstairs office, and went directly upstairs. Dragon Lady was not there. I wondered if I should be relieved at not having to deal with her or disappointed because there was no one to whom I could deliver my hard-won *solicitud*. In another office around the corner I found an associate of Dragon Lady. She was much friendlier, but correspondingly less powerful. She suggested that I simply take the paper directly to the president's office. That sounded OK to me.

The path to that august destination passed through another guarded gate and two more offices, each with its ever-watchful secretary. One finally accepted my petition, but said that *señor presidente* was out. He was to return around 4:30 that afternoon. I offered to stop by around 5:00. She looked dubious, but I smiled brightly and departed, still clutching my papers. However, at 5:00 P.M. I failed even to get through the downstairs gate. The soldier on guard did not remember me from the early afternoon. He said that the president was in a meeting with all of his staff, so I would have to call for a later appointment. "Call what person, at what number?" I pleaded. The guard didn't have any idea.

By this time I had nearly forgotten the actual boxes. The quest was taking on a life of its own. I returned home again.

At home, I received a note from Pam two weeks later. She had tried to make an appointment with the person whose name I had managed to glean from the downstairs reception office. It appeared that I was back to Square One. The person with whom I must meet was Dragon Lady herself. Ironically, her name turned out to be Socorro, a Spanish word meaning "help" or "assistance."

In the end, I was spared the ordeal of this face-to-face confrontation when someone from Explorama went there on my behalf and managed to officially unload the *solicitud*.

It was late November before I received word from Pam that the boxes had been freed. Her miraculous announcement coincided with the arrival of a post office notice in which I was informed that my four boxes, having sat unclaimed for almost three months, would shortly be Returned to Sender.

I rushed into the city. Once the papers had been put into an acceptable form, it appeared that presidential approval was nearly automatic. Further, in an astonishing display of cooperation, someone had telephoned Explorama's office with that news. We had simply to dispatch an Explorama employee to collect the documents. I retrieved the papers from Explorama and headed out to customs headquarters in Punchana, where I triumphantly presented the long-sought "Request from the Regional President for the Exoneration of Customs Duties." As I waited on their now-familiar bench, they typed up a form officially authorizing the exemption of duties and letting the post office know that they could hand over the loot.

From Punchana, I beat a hasty path to the post office in a bid to beat the early afternoon closing hour. I marched up the post office steps, breathless with the expectation that the boxes had been shipped home only yesterday. When that proved not to be the case, I offered the sheaf of papers which I held. They happily made the exchange, and I retreated to Explorama with all four boxes to sort them out and divide them into two equal piles so that I could fulfill my bargain with UTES.

That's why I tell people they cannot "send" medicines to me here.

CHAPTER NINE

# Fiesta

When people ask me what I miss most from my native country, I say, "My friends, my family, and my bike," the latter a 600 cc Kawasaki on which I have spent many pleasant and relaxing hours. To make up for the loss of my bike, I attend as many fiestas as I can, and dance. (Dancing is an activity—much like riding the bike—that I maintain is a reasonable substitute for sex, at least if you need a substitute. It would be nice to have the bike, sex, and rock 'n' roll, but then, life is never perfect.)

Fiestas are a major part of life here. People have no televisions, no bowling leagues, no tennis courts, few books to read. A fiesta may celebrate a hallmark in life such as a birthday or graduation, or it may mark a holiday (Catholic holidays and traditional Yagua holidays are celebrated with the same zest, and with the same rituals of drinking, dancing, and partying), or a fiesta may be held just for the fun of it.

One year, Juvencio's wife, Olga, invited me to her birthday celebration. I passed by the house in the afternoon, and the rafters were festooned with virgin white toilet paper, hand-stitched lengthwise down the center and gathered, this being the local version of crepe paper. Dozens of brightly colored narrow ribbons had been woven in and around and through the toilet paper and the rafters, dangling down in curls and swoops. In the center, where the toilet paper was pulled up to a peak, was suspended a white wedding bell of waffle-folded paper from Hallmark's Peruvian counterpart. The usual fishing net, hammock, tools, and child-generated debris had all been removed and the floor swept.

Back in the kitchen stood a thirty-gallon blue plastic garbage can filled with *masato*. This beverage, indispensable for any self-respecting fiesta in these parts, is made by boiling *yuca* roots. The boiled roots are chewed to a pulp by the women of the tribe and then allowed to ferment for a few days, the fermentation being initiated by the saliva of the masticators. Reputedly, the best *masato* is made by the eldest, most toothless women. I assume this is because they must chew longer to reduce the roots to a pulp, thus adding more of the fermenting saliva in the process. The resulting mass, at any rate, is mixed with water from the river to obtain the desired consistency, and is served in bowls. Its method of preparation aside, it has always looked, tasted, and smelled to me like wallpaper paste gone sour, and I turn it down on principle. But it has been the primary fuel for fiestas in this region since long before the people drinking it wore dresses or T-shirts.

Fortunately for me, the conquistadores brought the sugarcane plant with them when they arrived, about four hundred and fifty years ago. From this useful plant, a second inebriant is derived. It is manufactured at what is called, euphemistically, the rum factory, located at the junction of Yanamono Stream with the Amazon River. The cane, grown in the fields between here and there, is cut with machetes when ripe and taken to the *trapiche* (mill). The cane stalks are bludgeoned with a heavy stick to flatten their ends and fed into an ancient iron press, like a large wringer washer.

The resulting cane juice undergoes multiple fates. Some of it is drunk as is, a sort of jungle Kool-Aid. Some is allowed to ferment slightly on its own, becoming like a hard cider. Some is boiled all day in a large, shallow copper basin to produce *miel* (honey, otherwise known as sugarcane molasses). And some of it is put to ferment in hollowed-out logs that resemble dugout canoes.

The mash is eventually fed to the still, made of old oil barrels hammered flat and re-formed. From a small metal spigot at the base of the tank issues what can only be called a potent brew. Once I was offered a sample of the just-distilled product, and it was just like the old cowboy movies...take a cautious sip, swallow, and you suddenly grow hoarse and gasp for air, as your eyes bug out and steam vents from your ears. It is said to be up to 180 proof, though I imagine there is some variability, given the equipment used in its manufacture.

This brew is hauled to any social gathering in three- and five-gallon cans, hopefully to be diluted—although I have been at fiestas where, after nearly suffocating on a sip of the proffered beverage and gasping, "This isn't pure *trago*, is it?" I have been reassured: "Oh, no, *Doctora*, not at all—it's got sugar mixed with it!" (*Trago*, literally translated, means "drink," but the liquor's other name, *aguardiente*, means "burning water.")

The night of Olga's party, after having dinner and dressing up, I waited until around 9:00 or 9:30, when I could hear the distant roar of a portable generator being fired up, followed by the thrum of the base notes from the music. Then I took my flashlight and picked my way over the path (fortunately dry; I hate arriving with muddy feet) to their house. The usual procedure is to gather outside the house where the fiesta is taking place, to loiter for a while and decide if it's a good enough party to be worthwhile entering. True to form, there were knots of young men and a few young women clustered in the darkness just outside the fall of light from the house. I, being a friend, the *doctora*, a *gringa*, and an invitee, ascended the steps directly.

At the top of the steps, I was welcomed in by the beaming hostess. The room was brightly lit with the only electric light within many miles, this being an eighteen-inch fluorescent bulb suspended from a rafter and powered by the same generator that was chugging away back on the kitchen platform to provide electric current for the music. Outside the house, the darkness pressed close.

Clothing for the women varied from nice T-shirts and skin-tight Lycra shorts to fancy party dresses. Most women wore dresses, and all were painted with rouge, eyeshadow, and lipstick and had frilly decorations in their hair. The most common style of dress is form-fitting in the bosom, either sleeveless or with puffy sleeves, flaring out into layers of ruffles at the hips. These garments are made of brilliantly colored taffeta or satin and often garnished with lace and/or ribbons. For men, the usual garb is clean T-shirts in an amazing variety of logos, mostly of U.S. make and left by departing tourists. The other option is open-necked shirts in pale office stripes or in deep, vivid colors of challis. The T-shirts or long-sleeved shirts are worn over blue jeans or long pants. For footwear, men universally sport the kind of clumpy, bulky, ankle-high athletic shoes that make their feet look as if they comprise half the bulk of their legs, with the pants cuffs draped over the tops of their shoes as though the pants are too long for the legs filling them.

Children, as always, were scattered through the crowd. Baby-sitters are hard to come by, and besides, the *masato* is traditionally shared with any child old enough to drink from a bowl. Hammocks were strung in a couple of corners, with babies sleeping in them, oblivious. Later in the night, some of the smaller children would be sleeping on the floor beneath the benches, their older sisters warding off the mosquitoes with languid fanning movements. Against the wall between the *sala* and the sleeping area, just beneath the corner of the table bearing the stereo boombox and its speakers, sat Antonia, Juvencio's grandmother, a venerable old dame of eighty-some years, which is pretty advanced for here. She always sits on the floor, with her legs folded under her or stretched out in front, half smiling with her toothless mouth at the dancers, perhaps recalling other fiestas from days and nights gone by, when the music issued from flutes and drums and the party went on for days. She accepted the *masato* automatically when it came around.

After a while, a couple began to dance. The next song up, three or four others joined them, and after that, it was a free-for-all. By 11:00 P.M. or so, there were at least a hundred people in the twenty by thirty foot room, at least half of them dancing at any given moment. A couple of the Explorama guides have gone to the U.S. as guests of the various groups that have visited here, and when they come back, they always express puzzled amazement: "Everyone was wonderfully hospitable, and they treated me great, but when they held a big party for me, all we did was eat and talk, no dancing at all!"

Meanwhile, to keep the skids greased, Olga was circumnavigating the periphery, carrying an oft-refilled pitcher and a small tumbler. She would pause in front of each celebrant, pour, and offer the glass. This was *coktel*, a mixture of sugarcane rum, milk, beaten eggs, and vanilla. It tastes a lot like Bailey's Irish Cream, but is quite a bit stronger and will make short work of any inhibitions you may happen to have. Not that people here are especially inhibited. Everyone dances. The toddlers practice on the sidelines, moving their tiny hips with surprising fluidity. Men do not look shy and reluctant and mutter, "No, I'm sorry, I do not dance." Not hardly. In fact, they are sometimes more eager than their womenfolk, especially after the pitcher and bowls of *masato* have been around a few times.

On clear fiesta nights, I sometimes wander outside for a while to admire the starry sky or the moon or the strange silhouettes of the rainforest trees. The night of Olga's fiesta, it clouded up. It had been unusually dry and unusually hot for several weeks. That night, however, the stars abruptly disappeared, the night grew even blacker than usual, a strong wind suddenly blew through the proceedings, lightning flared and thunder boomed, and then the sky burst open and a wonderfully refreshing rain fell. It was a downpour at first and ran in glittering streams off the roof, where the thatch over-hangs the eaves of the house, and blew in on those of us who were on the side of the wind. Everyone who had been hanging around outside the front of the house came inside, and the already-packed floor filled even more densely.

I went back to the kitchen to hide from would-be dance part-ners and let the sweat dry for a bit in the cool breeze. The generator that ran the fluorescent light and the music box chugged noisily and odoriferously on the floor, and a hammock with a couple of small children in it swung gently in the center of the darkened kitchen. A steady brigade of girls old enough to be awake but still too young to be interested in boys came in, filled bowls at the plas-tic barrel of *masato*, gave the hammock a push to keep it moving, giggled to see me lurking in the shadows, and melted back into the hubbub in the main house. It was rather like watching a perfor-mance on a well-lit stage, from the vantage point of the darkness behind the curtains.

After a while, I dove back in. The pitch of excitement was still rising and would do so for quite a while yet. At midnight, the cake that had been baked in the lodge oven (none of the houses here have anything other than a cooking fire) was brought out. The music then halted, and the assembly was called to attention, not a difficult feat since everyone knew that (a) the music would not resume until this ceremony was completed and (b) the completion would entail the cutting and serving of the cake. A speech was offered in honor of the birthday celebrant, and the candles were then lit on the cake and blown out—multiple times since they were the kind that re-light themselves. Everyone joined in a spirited rendition of "Happy Birthday," sung to the same tune as the English version but with slightly different lyrics. I helped Olga cut the cake and took the pieces around the room, making sure that everyone got some.

The music then resumed, and the ball went on. I left not long thereafter ("So early, *Doctora*?!") When I passed the house the next morning on my way to open the clinic (and not till 9:00, either, it being a Sunday), there were still a few revelers on their feet and dancing, one or two more snoozed soundly on the benches or floor, and Juvencio sat, bleary-eyed but awake, with a large bottle of beer by his side. The party was a success.

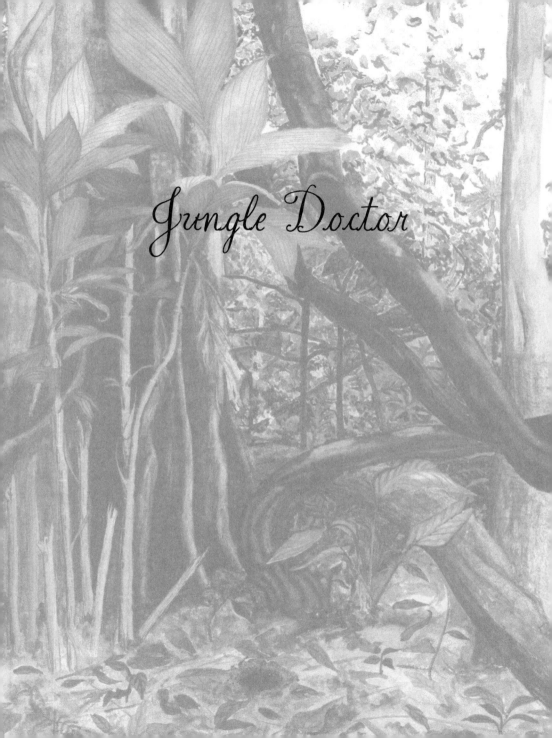

Jungle Doctor

# CHAPTER TEN

# Culture Clash

One of my favorite illustrations of the unpredictability of cultural differences comes from a story told by a Peruvian ecological worker. She and her associates were from Lima, but had been working with the people native to the high Peruvian jungle. This was more or less analogous, in U.S. terms, to a group of well-meaning and well-heeled Manhattanites setting out to help in Appalachia. The ecologists, at any rate, found that these particular people suffered from a diet severely deficient in protein.

The ecologists worked out a solution of which they felt they were justifiably proud: a method of raising capybaras, which are a sort of tailless giant beaver that weighs up to 120 pounds and provides a highly edible meat. The plan used simple corrals and locally available foodstuffs. It was a very ecologically sound idea, and easily within the technological and logistical grasp of the group it was to benefit. They then presented their proposal to the intended beneficiaries, only to be met with noncommittal stares. They explained, I imagine earnestly and with great enthusiasm, the many advantages of their system, but the response did not liven up at all.

It took a while for them to unearth the fact that these people believed that when their highly revered grandmothers died, they were promptly reincarnated as capybaras.

Oops.

Thus, "cultural differences" sometimes lie like traps in places where you don't even think to look for them. You can try to be culturally sensitive and pay attention to what others are doing—but how can you anticipate grandmother reincarnation?

Perhaps nowhere are the pitfalls of cultural differences felt more acutely than in the fields of medicine and religion, both of which touch people in the most intimate ways. I am no authority on religion, nor am I an ethnographer, but my work does bring me into contact with attitudes toward medical treatment.

For instance, a man from the Indian village across the stream, who had been afflicted by leishmaniasis for more than ten years, was not so confident in the benefits of modern medicine. Leishmaniasis, caused by a parasite transmitted by sand flies, affects the lining of the nose, and causes destruction of the nasal septum (the divider between the nostrils) and sometimes of the roof of the mouth. It also causes a gradual enlargement and flattening of the nose—all symptoms occurring slowly over a period of years. It isn't a common illness; the cases I've seen have been in hunters and healers, who ranged far into the forest for long periods of time.

When Absalom first came to see me, his nose was a wreck, and the disease was starting to invade his soft palate. He had seen a series of *brujos* over the years, but was resistant to the idea of modern therapy. I jumped up and down, stomped my feet, urged and practically threatened—he needed to go into Iquitos for treatment. Even though I assured him, multiple times over multiple visits, that I did not have the cure he needed, that both diagnostic testing and treatment were free, and that I would administer the injections at no charge, he never seemed to get around to making the journey. He dawdled, and he postponed, and he evaded, and he procrastinated. There was always a reason why he couldn't make the trip this week, and meanwhile the infection had spread to his larynx, making his voice hoarse, and was eating away at his palate.

He wanted penicillin, if he couldn't get antimony, and I had the problem of trying to explain that just any old antibiotic wouldn't do. By this time, the poor man looked miserable. His nose was ulcerating, and nearly the entire hard palate was involved.

He and his wife told me that they had gone to a hospital in Iquitos, he had been treated for fifteen days, and then he had been turned away for lack of money to pay for further treatment. It sounded a little odd, since the government program is free; when I went to the city myself, I could find no one in the program who had any record of this man as a patient. I confronted Absalom and his wife, and they hemmed and hawed and hedged.

Well, maybe it wasn't that hospital after all. Where had they gone, then? Oh, a private clinic. Name of clinic?—couldn't recall. Address of clinic?—couldn't recall. Name of doctor?—couldn't recall. Stalemate. I couldn't understand how they could be so vague, and from Yanamono I couldn't do much about it, nor was antimony available in any of the pharmacies I'd tried.

I had no choice but to let it lapse.

A month or so after this, they came once again, hoping that I had somehow been able to get hold of the antimony. I questioned them closely, but they stuck to the part about having received fifteen days of treatment. Now, however, they confessed that not only had the medicine not helped, it had actually made things worse. They had therefore gone to a *curandera* (healer), who had clarified that Absalom had been bewitched and that there was a devil residing in his nose. She performed the necessary rituals for casting out the devil and assured him that now when he received the medicine, not only would it do him no harm, but it would cure him. About the only part of their story that I was able to believe was the last segment about seeing the *curandera*. Absalom certainly could have had a reaction to antimony during fifteen days of treatment; however, their willingness to try it again, and even more, their evasiveness regarding just who had given it in the first place, made me suspect that all of their visits up until now had been to traditional healers.

I urged them as strongly as I could to (a) seek treatment in Iquitos immediately, through the Regional Hospital and (b) for heaven's sake, reveal the whole story of his treatment to date, to whomever wound up taking them on.

They went home, the clinic kept me occupied, and a couple of months passed. Then one day, while in the Yagua village, I realized I was near their house. I stopped beneath the raised floor and called up, "Hey, Absalom! Have you been yet for your treatment?" And, miracles abounding, yes, he had. I inquired as to his status—"better," he said. "Open your mouth," I said, and he did, and miracles remaining abroad in the land, the pebbly-looking area of the hard palate had improved considerably, now involving only about a third of the area that it had at its worst. What had he been taking? I wanted to know.

He pulled a former liquor bottle, nearly but not quite empty, from under the bench. He offered it for inspection. He invited me to sniff it. I detected sugarcane rum, the universal solvent, of course, and some leaves, of course. But what leaves? Can you describe the leaves? Oh, well, you know, he said, the ones the healer used.

OK, so how was this remedy applied? Ah, he said. I took two little cups (holding up a measure from a bottle of Pepto Bismol) on two separate days, he said. The medicine could not be consumed in the house, he added. It was necessary to walk into the jungle to take it, or it would be without effect.

But wait, I interjected. This is a one-liter bottle, and it's nearly empty. What happened to the rest of it?

Ah, he said. And he gestured, to illustrate. The rest of it, I rubbed through my hair, like this—combing with his fingers. And now I'm better.

And he was.

The biggest and most picturesque difference between modern medicine and most traditional medicine has to do with a basic difference in outlook. Modern medicine views illness as a clearly definable, frequently treatable set of occurrences confined to one human body, which in turn is composed of various physical parts and biochemical processes.

Traditional medicine in most cultures, on the other hand, tends to be more like a branch of religion than a branch of science and sees illness as a derangement involving a person and that person's relationship with the world in which he lives. Sometimes it even includes relatives, friends, and enemies. Lacking modern diagnostic methods and understanding of the physical and biochemical properties of human bodies, traditional conceptions of the nature of illness center around gods, spirits, witches, and other magical forces, which array themselves against someone and thus provoke physical and/or psychological symptoms. (And psychological symptoms are viewed, in this culture at least, in the same light as physical symptoms, so that, for example, failure to have the girl of your dreams fall in love with you is as much a problem needing "medicine" as is a fever and cough.)

The reasons for which a person is attacked by the various malevolent forces vary from one culture to another, but as far as I can tell, in this region illness is felt to be fairly random; that is, it is not usually that someone has offended the gods, or that some particular witch carries a grudge against the patient, but simply that someone, somehow, has become bewitched. In other parts of the world, efforts are made to determine who is the witching party and to demand recompense; as far as I know, that is not generally done in

Peru. The *brujo* simply announces that badness has been visited upon the sick person and determines that he will effect a cure.

The exceptions that I can recall are when the witcher was a dead relative. In one case, a little boy's diarrhea was explained as being due to his dead mother's efforts to induce him to join her, these efforts being instigated by her widowed husband's having taken a new wife who did not want her stepson. The child had been brought to me for diagnosis and treatment, but was also taken to the *brujo* for his contribution, a common situation: there is no need, here, to choose between "traditional" and "modern" medicine. The two co-exist, side by side, and covering all bases is felt to be a wise precaution. In the case of the boy, neither the shaman's medicine nor mine prevailed. The boy's dead mother eventually succeeded in her quest, probably helped along by the malnutrition that was at least partly attributable to her absence and the stepmother's indifference.

The belief that illness is caused by spirits obviously requires that the treatment be magical and be conducted with the patient's intimate involvement. Both the magic and the patient involvement are minimized in most modern medicine, although we do have our counterparts.

Technology is our magic; a CAT scan or blood test seem to most laypeople to be a necessary part of the cure, instead of the diagnostic procedures that they really are. Nonetheless, technology in general is a phenomenon with which we are familiar, which we use daily in the form of televisions, telephones, refrigerators, and so forth, and which therefore is at risk for being held in contempt. And the modern patient, although clearly involved in the treatment process, mostly becomes the nonparticipating subject of various maneuvers by physicians and other practitioners, with very little caretaking thrown in.

Traditional medicine, in contrast, does quite a lot of caretaking. Special diets are sometimes prescribed before treatment is even begun (this also provides an "out" for the *brujo* whose treatment fails: ah, it is said, the patient didn't follow the diet), other processes of purification such as abstinence from sex may be required, and the actual treatment process is likely to take place in a darkened room and to involve ritual and smoke and chanting and so forth, all of which serve to comfort and reassure the patient. It is this part of medicine, the caretaking process, that is lacking in modern medicine, and although most Westerners would find many shamanistic practices to be fairly untidy and occasionally downright distasteful, the idea of being hovered over is very appealing.

The benefit to this style of medical practice is that it is far more considerate of the entire person than the standard Western approach, which separates the person from the illness and treats the illness while often forgetting the person attached to it. In modern medicine, we usually underestimate the value of reassurance and empathy, whereas most of the traditional practices emphasize these all-important aspects of treatment.

Furthermore, at least some of the traditional medical practices also have validity in the Western sense. Most of our so-called modern medicines were derived from traditional ones, and there are surely many more potential medicines in use by traditional healers throughout the world.

There are some drawbacks to traditional medicine as well, however. Many of the physical ailments in the jungle, for instance, are bacterial in origin, and as far as I know, there are no really effective antibiotics among the *brujo*'s stores of knowledge. They do claim treatments for tuberculosis and have undoubtedly effective methods of birth control, treatment of warts, malaria cures—Peru is the home of the cinchona tree, a source of quinine—and there are some fairly promising compounds used to speed the healing of wounds. Many of these substances are currently under study by modern medicine in a field of research called ethnobotany. One of its goals is to find additional incentives to promote the preservation of the rain forest and of the many fast-disappearing cultures contained in it. Most of the remedies used by the *brujos* around here are not well-enough studied for me to feel comfortable using them, but I imagine that more of them will find their way into the realm of the known and may very well be part of my armamentarium in the future.

However, even the simplest recipes are being lost. When I asked a young woman from the Yagua village why she had not dosed herself with the sap of the oje tree, which purges intestinal worms, she replied that she did not know the correct dose to use.

Even worse, the knowledge that does still exist is inevitably becoming distorted and often replaced by home remedies that are a mixture of misinformation and misunderstanding—as in the case of the woman who blithely rubbed DDT into the open sores on her young child's body because a well-meaning neighbor told her it was the thing to do. (In fact, that treatment probably would have been excellent had the problem been a botfly, but that was not what the child had.) This problem is multiplied manyfold by the ready availability of medicines. Virtually any medicine can be bought simply by going into any pharmacy and paying for it. Prescriptions are not needed, even for powerful antibiotics and injectable drugs. This engenders a good deal of inappropriate self-treatment, as well as promoting conditions in which bacterial resistance can arise, so that the bacteria causing illness become immune to the medicines used to treat them—an even more common, and deadly, problem in the United States, where we use immense amounts of antibiotics.

And, of course, this is all complicated even further by the cultural differences between a Wisconsin *gringa* and the people living here, who are caught in the throes of Westernization of what was never before a Western-style culture. These cultural differences affect not only expectations of treatment, but equally important, the manner in which illness and even anatomy are viewed.

For example, a man came one day with a bite from a poisonous snake. I tended to that problem (the bite was already several days old, and he was improving anyway); then as he was leaving, apparently almost as an afterthought, one of his family members asked me,

"*Doctora*, what about *mal dormido*?" "*Mal dormido*?" I echoed—bad sleeping? I assured them that he should be able to sleep just fine, but that if he had trouble, he could take the pain medicine I had supplied. They nodded politely and left. Wondering, I asked one of the guides if *mal dormido* had any particular significance in the setting of a snakebite. And, I learned, it surely does. There exists a belief that if someone has been bitten by a snake and someone else in the house engages in sexual activity while the healing process is still underway, then the person bitten will fail to heal properly and may even die. So much for my cheery reassurance that he should be able to sleep well.

Another day, a young man who lives nearby came to request a house call for his wife, who had given birth a few days earlier. I discourage house calls whenever possible, to avoid keeping other patients waiting at the clinic and to avoid the difficulties of trying to treat in the local homes. This patient did not sound too sick to walk the short distance from her house to the clinic, so I suggested that she come here instead of me going there. He protested that she was unable to leave her bed, not for reasons of weakness, but because she had not yet fulfilled the prescribed eight days of rest following a birthing. While this mandated rest may not be medically necessary, the tradition has my support because it is the only opportunity these poor women ever have to rest from cooking, hauling water, washing clothes, tending babies, and doing all their other tasks. However, I explained that if she was ill, I could care for her much more ably in my cubbyhole than in hers. He continued to argue for a house call, saying she was bleeding from the delivery, and therefore must be broken inside. I tried to clarify that nothing was actually "broken" and that the bleeding following childbirth was more like a big menstrual period.

He pondered this for a minute or two. Then he said, diplomatically, "Well, *Doctora*, that probably is true in your country. But your society is much more advanced than ours, so your bodies are probably very different!"

Then there is the universal admiration for "shots." This, I think, is a consequence of the fact that the first antibiotics, which must have made a huge splash, were always injectable; in addition, there is an eagerness to adopt Western ways, which makes any fragment of technology irresistibly appealing. At any rate, from barely past infancy, everyone here KNOWS that if you are really ill, only a shot will cure you. Oh sure, pills and tonics are OK if it's a minor illness, but if the illness is serious, then a shot is obviously, indubitably, inarguably, and urgently called for.

Sometimes, when people come into the clinic and I ask them what they need today, they tell me solemnly, "I need a shot." When someone comes hoping for an injection and I prescribe medicine to be taken orally, often the person listens attentively to my explanation as to why the pills are superior in effect to the requested shot, nodding his or her head in obedient acquiescence. Then when I hand over the medication, I hear, "But when do I get my shot?"

This insistence on being stuck with a needle stems from a variety of reasons. Many times a neighbor or *sanitario*, one of the first-aid workers most small villages have, has recommended this mode of treatment; or a friend may recently have had "just the same illness" and received an injection, and they'd like to get what the friend had, please. On occasion, I think it's just the pretty color of the medicine that appeals. (In the early days, when there was no separate pharmacy room and all the medicines were in one open cabinet, people would occasionally peer into the cabinet and say, "Oh, that's an interesting-looking pill—could I have some of those, please?" without the least idea of what the medicine was for).

And, of course, the element of drama is not to be discounted in a society tending toward the hypochondriac in the first place. Here, where the technology is not available for such heroics as resuscitation or MedFlight, "needing an injection" conveys the gravity of the situation.

Once, it was reported to me that the popular local schoolteacher was deathly ill. I had recently seen her for what sounded like hayfever, and evidently this had progressed to a terrible cough preventing her from sleeping at night, with great difficulty in breathing, high fever, and so on. She was, according to my informant, in desperate need of an *ampolla* (literally, an ampule of medicine, i.e., an injection). When I arrived at her home, entered her room, and pulled aside the mosquito netting, I found her looking a bit tired but otherwise healthy. She smiled at me bravely and gave a small, phlegmy-sounding cough. Her skin was dry and not feverish, her color was normal, her breathing not rapid, her lungs clear when I listened with my stethoscope, and she was not wheezing. OK, so maybe she had a touch of bronchitis. That does not necessarily produce dramatic physical signs, but it is nonetheless an illness, and a treatable one. I murmured reassurances and promised to return immediately, bearing *remedios*.

A concerned friend dogged my steps anxiously on the walk in to the lodge. He asked me urgently about the *ampolla*. No, no, I reassured him. I had excellent and potent medicine to treat her with, I explained, but I didn't think there was an *ampolla* that would help her. The antibiotic I had in mind, in oral form, was quite a bit stronger than the penicillin that was the only antibiotic I had available for injection. He remained unconvinced, knowing that no matter what this *gringa* might say, everyone KNOWS that an *ampolla* is more powerful than pills, any day.

I duly delivered the drugs, carefully explained how to take them, and promised to check back the following day.

The next morning, the man pounced on me even before breakfast. The *maestra* (teacher) was no better, he pronounced, in deeply worried tones. She had passed a terrible night, could hardly breathe, practically died, and really NEEDED an *ampolla*.

And he had just the thing, purchased yesterday in Iquitos, where news of the dire situation had been relayed urgently by radio. He conveyed that they did not hold it against me that I was incapable of coming up with a cure, but that it was now taken care of. All they needed from me was to administer the lifesaving stuff, which was guaranteed to work infallibly in "cases like this"—just the very thing for breathing difficulties. Arriving at the sickbed, I again found my patient in no distress whatsoever that I could see. Once again, her bedside was guarded by a gallant admirer. Once again, her lungs were clear and she had no fever.

I asked for the *ampollas*, and they were promptly and reverently brought out. There were three, prescribed by an Iquitos pharmacist who had not laid eyes on the patient. I examined them. Two of the vials, about five cc each (a goodly quantity of liquid to inject) contained a fluid of a very pretty shade of bright emerald green. I could discover no labeling at all on one of them, but its twin still bore a few faint letters indicating that it was oil of eucalyptus. These were to be given, according to the prescribing pharmacist, one today, the other tomorrow morning. The remaining ampule was to be administered tomorrow evening. It was lincomycin, a decent but rather outmoded and not particularly potent antibiotic, of which one dose would accomplish little or nothing anyway. I assumed (not without misgivings), since the green potion had been sold by a pharmacy, that it was at least meant (however unadvisably) for injection into human beings, and should not kill her. The premier rule of medicine is "First, do no harm," and this injunction made me hesitate to administer that which I knew was at best useless. On the other hand, her many concerned friends would see to it that sooner or later she got injected with something, and if I didn't do the deed now, with the means currently in my hand, someone else would proceed— very possibly using even worse substances than what I then held. I pulled out a syringe and swabbed one smooth hip with a cotton ball doused in perfume, the only form of alcohol in the house other than sugarcane rum. The ostensibly lifesaving green solution was thick and syrupy, but I eventually got it injected. Then I crossed my fingers, hoping that whatever it was that I had just given, it would not prove to be fatal…an anaphylactic reaction would be a terrible price to pay for the comfort of a green placebo. I did succeed in getting the patient's friends to agree to hold off on the other ampules.

Then I left, shaking my head.

I didn't hear any more of her for quite a while. Months later, word filtered back that she had been slow to improve. Her attentive circle of supporters, eager to help, sought and obtained one injection after another, until finally one of them left an abscess that gouged a sizable hole in her backside.

All in the name of health. Although in my native, ostensibly more "developed," country, we pursue some fairly dubious courses of treatment ourselves—and ours cost quite a bit more.

# CHAPTER ELEVEN

# Necrotizing Fasciitis

I can say, without need for false modesty, that I am the best physician for miles around. Of course, I could say equally truthfully that I am the worst, but I don't because it doesn't have quite the same ring to it. The main reason that I am the best, the worst, and the average is that I am the only. The nearest other doctor is at Indiana, and I have already touched upon the limitations of the care available there, not to mention the fact that transport to the *posta* is not always available or affordable. My patients are poor people, for whom the ten or twenty dollars necessary to buy passage and food for the patient and a family member may be an unobtainable sum. Then there would be the additional costs of the treatment itself.

At Pevas, another hundred miles or more downriver, there is a *posta* similar to the one at Indiana. Or a twenty-two-and-a-half-hour journey from Mazan, a town on the Napo River to which one can walk from Indiana, will bring you to the mission town of Santa Clothilde, where a group of Franciscan missionaries has a well-equipped small hospital. And there is the Iquitos hospital itself, essentially an oversized version of Indiana, with many of the same problems of supply and materials—if, again, you can get there at all in the moment of your need.

As a result of these logistical realities, my patients come from a fairly large geographical area. About six hours of travel seems to be the limit, depending on the nature of the problem. While few people would travel that distance for minor illnesses, someone might indeed walk over from the village across the stream for a simple runny nose. Conversely, the farther people have had to travel, the more likely they are to be seriously ill, and the more likely they are to have brought friends, relatives, and neighbors along, since the journey is being made anyway—might as well get everyone in for treatment all at once.

One Sunday morning, I heard footsteps coming up the front stairway and into the waiting area. Going out to check, I found a middle-aged woman lying on her back on the floor, her panting family standing around her, and the hammock in which they had carried her arrayed around her supine body. They had come from a small village over on the Napo River, and I never did find out how they had traveled. If they had arrived by *colectivo* (river taxi), they would have been en route for a minimum of eight hours. The journey through the forest on foot takes three-and-a-half hours for a healthy, quick walker; heaven only knows how long it must have taken if they were carrying her in the hammock the whole way.

The problem, they explained, was a "tumor" of the lady's private parts, which would not permit her to sit down. It had been present for a somewhat indeterminate length of time—maybe a week. Maybe two. I expected to find either a prolapsed uterus (the uterus, surrendering to gravity after the strain of having borne eight or ten children, simply loses its footing in the lower abdomen and slides down through the vagina—not a life-threatening problem, but if it gets to the point where the organ is actually dragging on the seat of the chair every time you sit down, it can be a real nuisance) or an advanced uterine or cervical cancer. Once we had carried her to the exam room and lifted her up onto a table (she was in too much pain to walk even that far), I found she had a fever of 104 degrees and cellulitis involving her entire perineum. "Cellulitis" should not be confused with "cellulite," the term popular among dieters to describe the loose fat draped around their thighs and tummies. Cellulitis is a medical term for infection of the soft tissues, that is, the skin and the underlying fat and/or connective tissue—a far worse problem to have than cellulite. "Perineum" is the medical term for the external genitals and their immediate environs, or in slightly less medical terminology, the crotch. Hers was red, swollen, hot to the touch, and obviously quite painful. The vulva on the right was especially swollen, but I could not locate any soft spots that would have indicated areas where the tissues were liquefying and could be opened and drained. (If there are such areas, they must be opened, or else, as with an abscess, you can take antibiotics until the sloth comes home, but the thing won't heal, because the antibiotics cannot penetrate the dead tissue.)

Although the entire area looked awful, no part of it was yet ready to be drained. Technically it was still a cellulitis and might, with luck, be amenable to antibiotic therapy. Accordingly, I gave her ciprofloxacin—the grown-up version of penicillin—a tremendously potent antibiotic that should cure practically any bacteria alive, on a body or in it. The following day, her left side was just a little less red, a little less swollen, a little less hot, and she didn't have to stifle a scream when I examined her. The right side, however, was even more ugly than it had been on Sunday morning. I still couldn't find an incipient opening, so injected a bit of local anesthesia, probed around inside with a needle and syringe, and withdrew a tiny amount of purulent material—pus, in English. I added metronidazole, another antibiotic, useful against anaerobic bacteria, the bugs who live where light and air never penetrate.

The next morning, a small, irregular patch of necrotic skin appeared on the right side. In a two-and-a-half by three-and-a-half centimeter area, the skin was black and dry and looked like the skin on a pumpkin left out in the first really hard frost. I gently trimmed it off, and out flowed two or three tablespoons of indescribably foul-smelling material, not your good old garden variety yellow stuff that you can get out of any simple abscess, but a thick gray soup of melted flesh that would have made Edgar Allen Poe feel right at home. The smell lingered at the back of my palate all day, no matter how many times I washed and bathed and brushed my teeth. I scraped out all the dead and dying tissue that I could, in an attempt to reach the clean base underneath. However, the infection had progressed from a simple cellulitis to what would be called necrotizing fasciitis. "Necrotizing," simply enough, means "dying." Not the patient, with a little luck, but the tissues composing the patient; although of course if sufficient tissue dies, the person cannot be too far behind. Small amounts of necrotic tissue are routinely seen in such minor problems as pimples. Fasciitis, however, has much wider implications.

The human body is not composed of a uniform jelly contained in a bag of skin. Rather, it is made up of bones, internal organs, muscle, fat, and so on. These components are held in place by ligaments and other connective tissues, forming compartments in the body. The fascia is the layer of tough fibrous tissue that separates these compartments from one another. When you cut into a piece of steak and encounter a silvery sheet of fibers that cannot be cut with a fork, you have found fascia. Normally, if you have cellulitis, the fascia prevents the infection from going deeper and entering the muscle. If an infection actually does get into the muscle, the next layer of fascia prevents it from spreading to the next deeper compartment.

Unless the fascia itself becomes infected. In that case, the infection can follow the fascial plane and run wild through the body, as a fire would race through the walls of a house.

Since it is impossible to "cure" dead tissue and since the dead tissue serves as a center from which infection spreads outward, the treatment of necrotizing fasciitis involves not only the use of antibiotics to control the infection at its advancing front, but also removal of all the dead material. In the manner of a back burn to

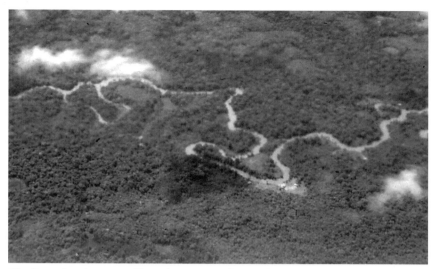

The Peruvian Amazon. Note the many twists and cutbacks caused by constant erosion of the banks.

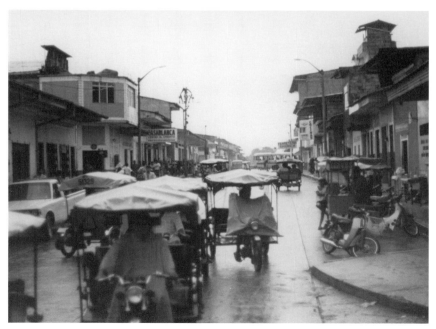

*Motokars,* motorcycles whose back wheels are replaced by small covered coaches, serve as taxis in downtown Iquitos, Peru.

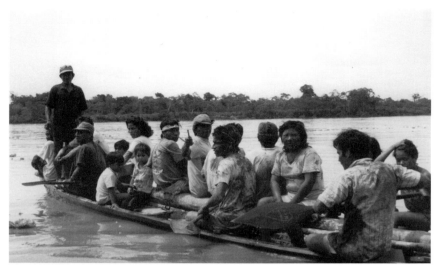

Yagua villagers travel in an open boat powered by a long-tailed motor called a peki-peki.

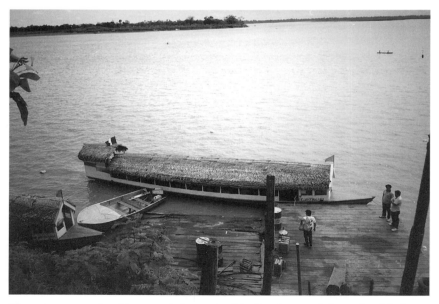

The primary mode of transportation out of Iquitos (up- and downriver) is by *pamacari*, a thatch-roof boat. Note the open-air outhouse behind the motor.

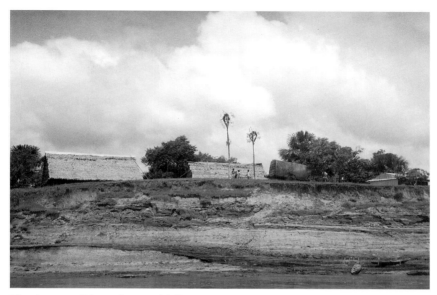

The Amazon River rises and falls up to 35 feet each year. During low-water season, makeshift steps cut into the steep clay banks allow access to the village.

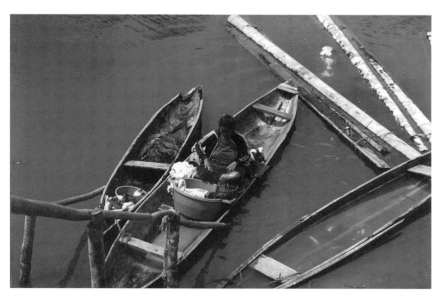

A woman in a dugout canoe washes clothes in the river.

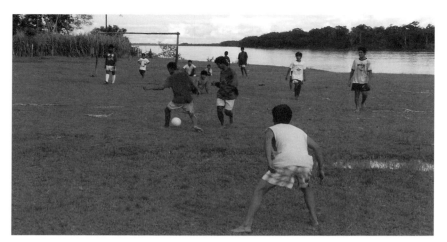

*Futbol* (soccer) is the unofficial national sport of Peru. Playing fields can be found in even the smallest villages.

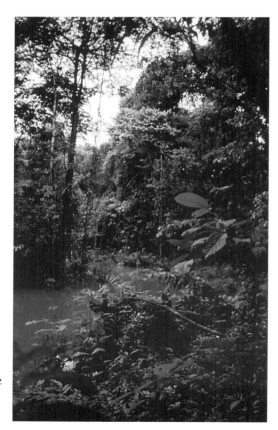

A path through the jungle

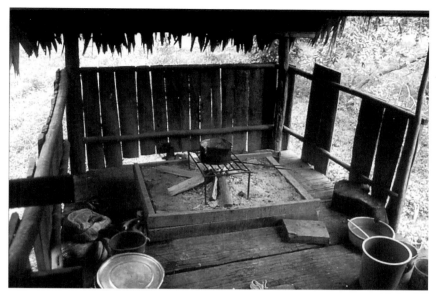

Cooking takes place over an open fire in a room attached to the house. The hearth is called a *tushpa*.

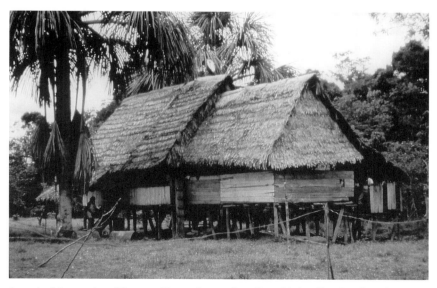

A typical house in a Yagua village sits on five-foot-high stilts. During the rainy season, water rises to just below the floorboards.

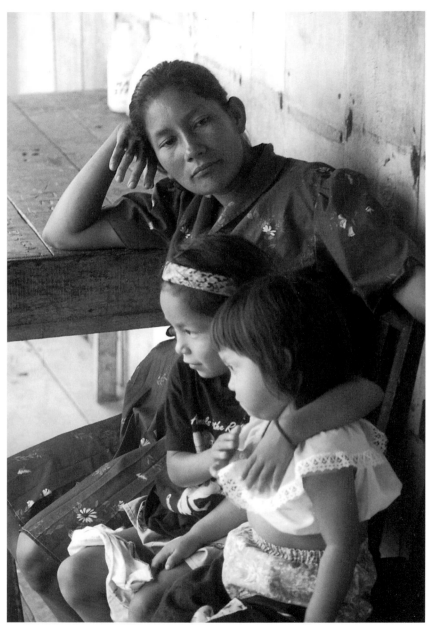

A woman and her children in the waiting room of the original Clínica Yanamono.

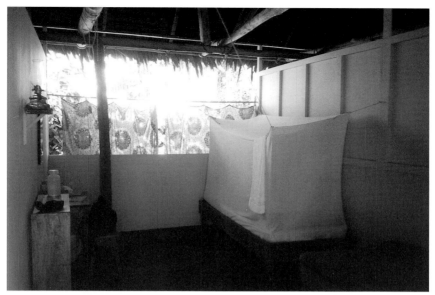

A guest room at Explorama Lodge. The unscreened half-wall opens out onto the jungle, so mosquito nets drape over every bed. Light is provided by kerosene lamp.

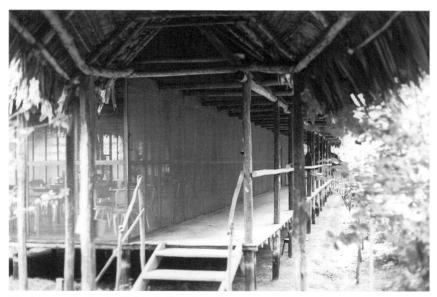

Explorama Lodge's dining hall and walkway

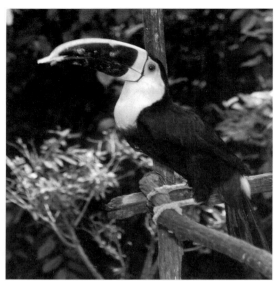

A Couvier's Toucan

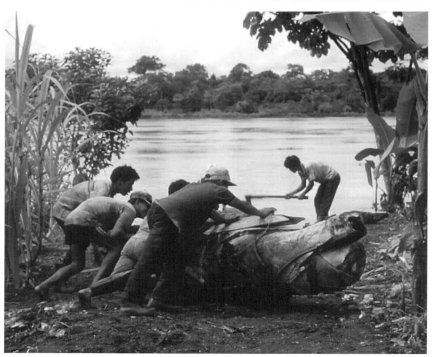

A group of men transform a large tree trunk into a dugout canoe.

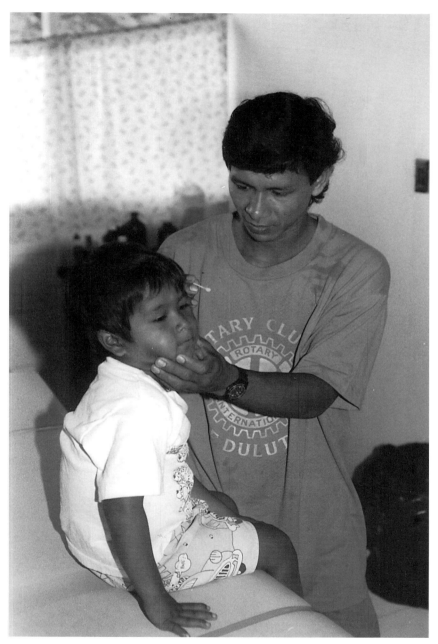

Juvencio examines a young patient.

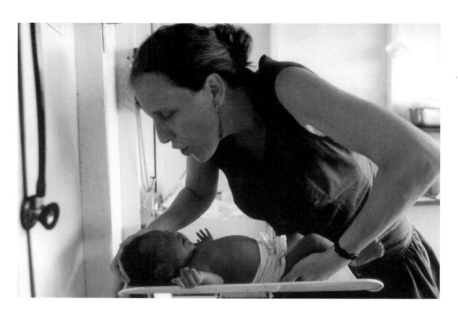

Approximately two-thirds of the people seen at the Yanamono clinic are adults.

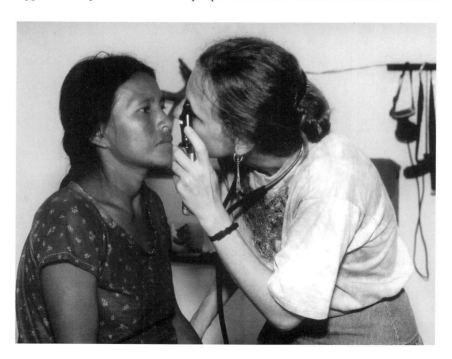

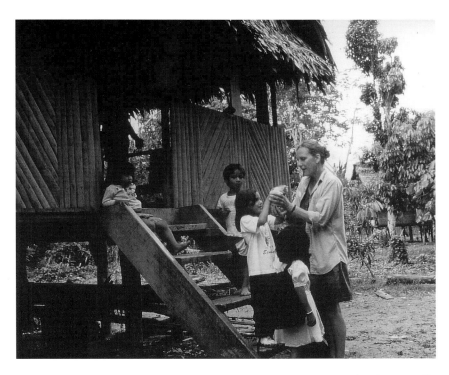

Even with the new clinic complete, Linnea still occasionally makes house calls.

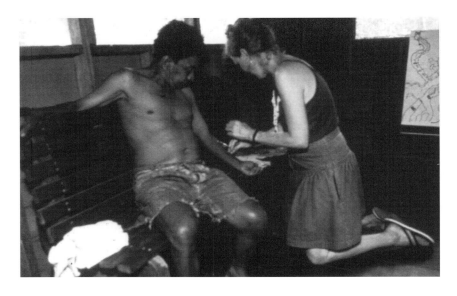

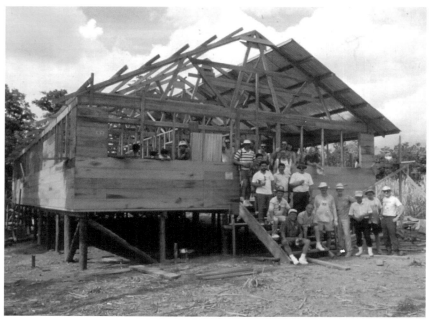

Construction crews from the Duluth, Minnesota, and Thunder Bay, Ontario, Rotary clubs pose on the steps of the new clinic facility.

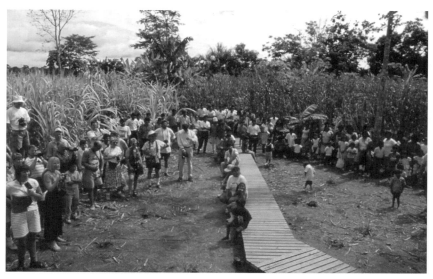

Opening Day!

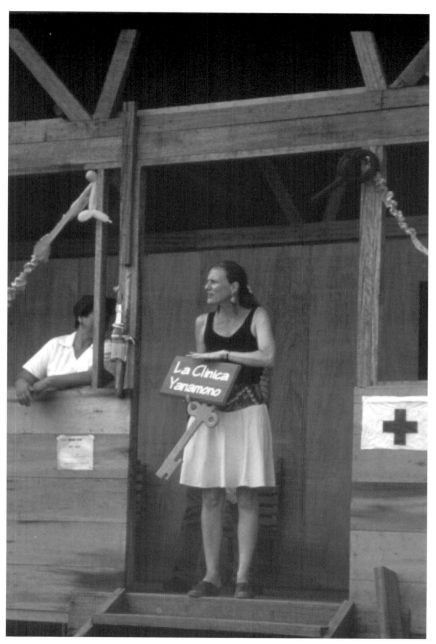

Linnea accepts the clinic's key at a dedication ceremony.

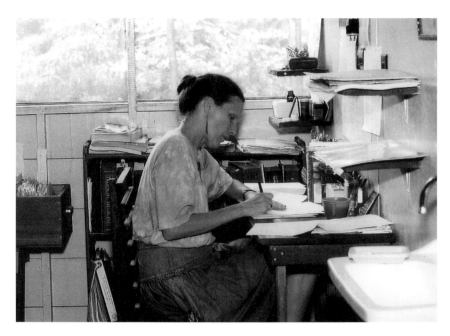

Linnea's office and an examination room in the new clinic.

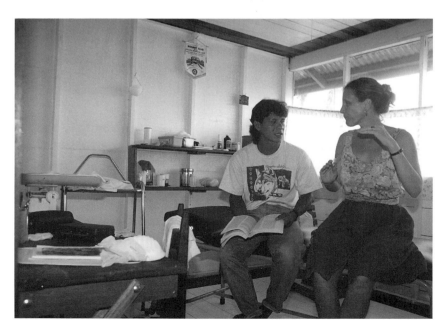

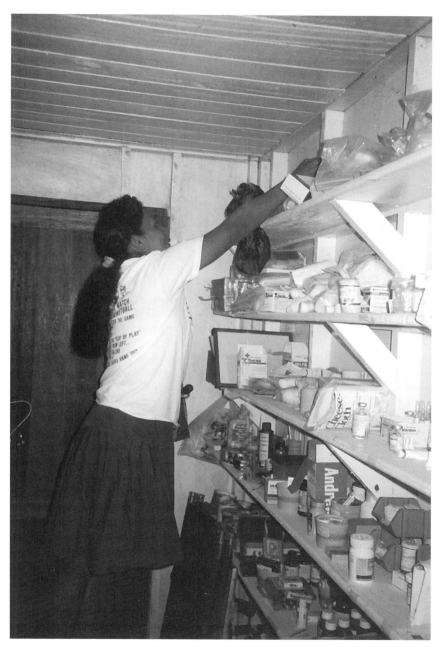

The new pharmacy

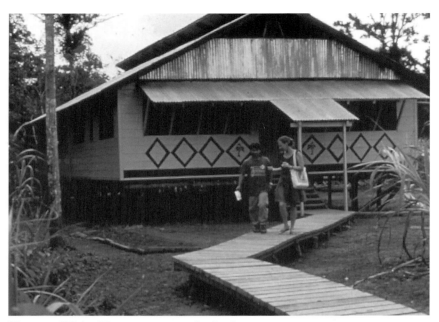

The new Clínica Yanamono opens for business

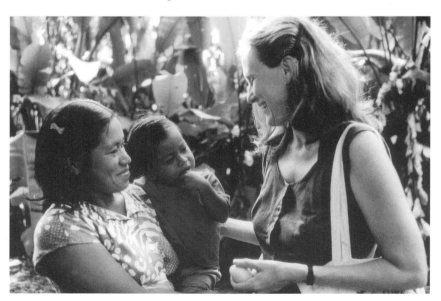

Sincere appreciation to Jon Helstrom, Dan and Judy Peterson from the Amazon Medical Project, Karl Nollenberger and Moonshadow Photography for the use of their photographs.

control a fire, this removal must include not only ALL of the dead tissue, but usually a margin of apparently healthy flesh as well, to assure that the bacteria are not already invisibly at work in what still appears to be normal tissue. This type of surgery is called wide excision, because that's exactly what is done. A wide area is cut out, in order to assure that the antibiotics can penetrate all that is left. The patient can hardly win. Either the infection itself leaves a huge defect (again, in English, a gaping hole—the kind of infection typified by the "carnivorous streptococcus" that so recently terrorized the world) or the surgery leaves equally large gaps. And therein lay the problem. This could easily turn into major surgery. I well remembered, from my medical student training in reconstructive plastic surgery, that in cases involving the removal of large blocks of necrotic tissue from people's bodies, the damage never, ever turned out to be less extensive than what we had anticipated. We had often ended up plumbing into depths that I didn't even want to think about out here in the wilds, far from adequate IV fluid, sterile operating conditions, and, especially, extra hands.

The following morning, the poor woman clambered yet again up onto the table for examination. My clinic assistant, Juvencio, held the light and handed me gauze and iodine as I probed gently. The left side was responding to the antibiotics and appeared slightly but noticeably improved. But her right vulva was now swollen all the way up to her abdomen, at least five or six inches farther than it had been the previous evening. The area where I had removed the blackened skin had opened up into a tunnel that ran backward into her buttock. I inserted my gloved finger, and it slid under the skin up to my knuckle. The only reason it stopped at that point was that the knuckle was attached to the rest of my hand, which could not enter. Yet.

She needed an incision twelve to fifteen inches long, with removal of a pound or so of flesh. At the least.

It goes without saying that her family was quite poor. In any case, there were no boats bound that day for Iquitos, where at least she could have gone to a real hospital with a real operating room and at least a few nurses and therapists to help with her recovery. So I opted for Indiana. We loaded her and two family members into the small clinic boat, and off we went.

Once there, we found we were in luck—the doctor was in, which is not always the case. However, he did not appear to feel that it was a good day for me to be bringing him a patient of this sort. He evidently had had a busy morning, because he was shirtless when we arrived, during what should have been his lunch hour. He did not respond to my explanations with unbridled enthusiasm.

As an alternative to surgery, he suggested irrigating the area with drains, or rubber tubes, followed by heavy-duty antibiotics. Again, I bit my tongue—they'd never go for it at the University of Wisconsin. But I was, after all, on his turf, and asking his help. I could hardly order him to tailor that help to my ideas of what should be done.

So that was what we did. He gave the woman a local anesthetic, used a long forceps to slide several lengths of flexible tubing into the tunnels opening up under her skin, and washed the area with copious amounts of sterile irrigating fluid. I left money with him to cover the cost of the antibiotics, because her family could not have paid for the medicine, and headed home.

On the way, I contemplated whether or not I should have taken the more aggressive tack myself at Yanamono. The advantage of the Peruvian physician's approach, if she recovered, would be much less scarring and a shorter recovery time than if she had undergone extensive surgery. The disadvantage was a smaller likelihood of recovery, and a rather grim manner of dying if she failed to recover.

She did recover, however—a testimony to the resilience of the human body, and equally a testimony to the validity of low-tech, simple methods of medical care and to the wisdom of this doctor's approach.

In the United States, I think we are sometimes more aggressive in our treatment than we truly need to be. It is very difficult to know in advance the best course to take. If I had operated at Yanamono and she had died, I would have felt horrible; if I had operated and she had recovered, I would have felt certain that that would have been the only possible hope for her and would have done it that way again the next time. Now, the next time I see a patient like this, I too will insert drains.

CHAPTER TWELVE

# Tropical Diseases

I am often asked about the prevalence of esoteric, exotic, or down-right weird diseases here, and also about my own health.

As for exotic diseases, there are a few, of course. I very rarely had to treat piranha bites or freshwater stingray injuries when I was in Wisconsin (although neither of those problems is exactly run-of-the-mill here, either). There have been a few cases of cholera, which can be a bad disease, though fortunately a short-lived one ("short-lived" referring to the illness itself, not to the patient, at least not usually). And after years of quiescence, malaria has made its reappearance in the neighborhood. I have also seen a handful of cases of leishmaniasis, a disease caused by microscopic parasites that take up residence in the lining of the nose and throat and, gradually over a period of years, erode those structures away.

One of the tricky things about practicing medicine here is that I occasionally encounter diseases that have become obsolete in the U.S. I have also fumbled my way around, treating a few exotic diseases for which my only training was long-forgotten lectures way back in medical school. In both cases, I have been treated to a few lessons in "jungle medicine."

Consider, for instance, tuberculosis. It remains, despite its recent comeback, a relatively uncommon disease in the United States. So, my own experience with tuberculosis, and with the medicines used to treat it, was theoretical, not practical.

During my first months here, before I was fluent in Spanish, a man named Adolfo from the Yagua village came by one day asking for medicine for tuberculosis. I tried to explain to Adolfo that he needed to go to the tuberculosis program in Iquitos, where the testing was performed and medication supplied free of charge. He kept insisting on pills, and I kept reiterating that I had none for tuberculosis.

A few days later he returned with a vial of streptomycin powder, the sterile water with which to reconstitute it, and the request that I inject him with the mixture. The guide translating for me that day told me that Adolfo had had tuberculosis since his early twenties (that would have been thirty to thirty-five years, more or less, though the man himself was rather fuzzy on his exact age). Apparently, he had been treated in the past for tuberculosis, but when or how adequately, it was impossible to know. At some undefined point in time, according to my translator, Adolfo had resumed smoking, drinking, and messing around with women, and his illness had therefore returned.

I attempted to explain to my translator that none of the activities in question could engender nor promote tuberculosis, but the patient had evidently been advised to abstain, so the guide and I had a brief digression in English on that subject, which I asked him to pass along to the would-be patient. Something was evidently lost in the translation, however, because several weeks later I was told by a third person that Adolfo's confidence in me had been severely shaken because I had advised him to build a platform high in a tree, climb up there, and remain for six weeks, completely avoiding alcohol, tobacco, and women for that interval.

At the moment, however, here he was on my doorstep, demanding to be injected with streptomycin, a medicine that should not be used lightly, as its side effects include kidney damage and loss of hearing, both permanent. I got the impression that he had had fifteen days of treatment with streptomycin administered by a friend, but that wasn't clear. Nor was it clear how long it had been since his last treatment, nor whether he was taking other medications, although it did seem that he was not currently on oral medication, which meant he was probably not enrolled in the government's tuberculosis program. Then again, who knew? Based on this surfeit of information, I had to decide which was the lesser of two evils: risk treating him unnecessarily (the only evidence of disease was the man's conviction that he had it) or risk not treating him when he really did have tuberculosis, which in fact is so endemic among the Yaguas as to make it quite likely that he did have the disease. I sighed and reconstituted the streptomycin. As I was about to inject it into one of his skinny hips, he intercepted me in alarm. Looking at the syringe with widened eyes, he told our translator that there were supposed to be five doses in the bottle, not just one.

I sheepishly squirted four-fifths of the liquid back into its vial, gave him the remaining two cubic centimeters, and instructed that he return on the morrow.

He was absent several days, then reappeared one evening. This time around, it appeared that Adolfo did not want an injection. Not from me, anyway. He wanted his vial of medicine. He intended to take it back to his village, where his friend, who had evidently only been on temporary leave, had returned. It seemed he was convinced that I had given him far too high a dose the first time, he had suffered terribly and had nearly died in the night, and he preferred to return to his acquaintance for the balance of his treatment.

I concluded that I needed to learn more about streptomycin and about the regimen used hereabouts for treating tuberculosis.

There was also the famed cholera epidemic that swept through South America in the early nineties, although it was never the scourge that the newspapers made it out to be. Cholera is an uncomfortable disease while you have it, and it has killed many thousands of people over the centuries. But most of those deaths could have been avoided by a few simple measures. Cholera is prevented by drinking clean water; that is, by not drinking other people's sewage. This of course is why it rarely affects tourists and always hits hardest in the very poorest areas of the countries where it is occurring. It is also a treatable disease. Cholera does not cause fever, the illness produces no toxic effects on the body, and it lasts only three or four days. Death, when it occurs, is caused by dehydration, as cholera provokes a watery diarrhea that can result in the loss of as much as fifteen or twenty liters of fluid a day. That can be one quarter of a person's whole body weight. Dehydration develops rapidly and can be severe enough to kill. Treatment, therefore, is simple: give fluids. If begun early, fluid replacement can usually be accomplished by mouth, although intravenous rehydration becomes necessary if the disease is allowed to progress. The problem is that among the people here, especially the less sophisticated ones, the idea is that you stand around and do nothing until the patient is on the verge of death, then you make a dash for the doctor.

And it is a messy disease, with fishy-smelling water issuing from the patient at alarming speed. One man was brought in and dumped unceremoniously on the clinic's doorstep when he was taken ill while traveling to Iquitos by river taxi. He was fifty-six years old and had been minding the family fields while his wife and children were all in Iquitos. Since he was bachelorizing, of course he didn't bother to boil the river water before drinking it.

I wasn't at the clinic when the man arrived, since there was then a shortage of intravenous fluid and I had gone to the city to try to find more. Such shortages do not occur in the United States, where a shortage of intravenous fluid would be comparable to a shortage of milk—it simply does not happen. Here, however, supply lines to the world outside the rain forest are tenuous, and I cannot always find the medicines I need in Iquitos.

I returned from the city, to find a worried Juvencio tending this extremely sick patient. He had already given the man four or five liters of fluid intravenously, and the fellow was still without a measurable blood pressure. He could not be given oral fluids; once a person reaches a certain point of dehydration, everything taken by mouth comes right back up, and rehydration must be intravenous until the person can again tolerate liquids by mouth.

I had succeeded in finding a few liters of fluid in Iquitos, and we gave the man one of those liters. His blood pressure came up a little, but by late afternoon, his eyes were still quite sunken, his skin was wrinkled like a well-dried prune, and, although we had given him a total of six-and-a-half liters of liquid—over a gallon and a half—he had lost more than four liters just in the clinic, plus who knew how much more in the boat on the way in. I decided to stay the night. By 8:00 P.M., his blood pressure was again too low to detect with the stethoscope, his eyes were rolling back in his head, and he was now complaining of a diffuse pain in the abdomen.

By 10:00 P.M. that night, I estimated his odds for survival at less than 10 percent. I had seen other patients with cholera, and they all look bad, but this man looked really bad. However, I had a difficult decision to face: Could I afford to give the little remaining fluid that we had to this man, who looked likely to expire at any minute? Or should I save it for another patient, who might or might not come in—perhaps another patient with cholera, or a woman hemorrhaging after childbirth, who might be saved by a liter of fluid? Did I say, enough is enough, save the remaining three liters for the next emergency, and just stand around and watch this man die? In the end, I gave him one more liter, slowly, stretching it out as much as possible. His luck finally kicked in, and he improved a little; by morning he was able to take a little fluid by mouth, and he wound up surviving. But I hate having to make those kinds of decisions.

I also once attended to an older man who had had a whole-body itch for seven years and had been to any number of healers, herbalists, and "doctors in the marketplace," but never to a physician. His skin, from neck to toe but worsening noticeably lower down, was thickened, scaly, dry, and obviously much scratched-at. At his ankles the skin was so thickened, it was like an elephant's. When he improved only slightly with the steroids I first tried, I took a biopsy and sent it to my friends in the U.S. (having long since learned that biopsies sent to Lima might as well have been sent to Luna). The results came back: "many neurotropic (nerve-seeking) acid-fast bacilli"—or in laypeople's terms, leprosy.

None of these so-called "tropical" diseases are exactly common, however. Far more common are prosaic diseases—diarrhea, pneumonia, malnutrition—which don't look much different from the same diseases in the U.S., but which occur with much higher frequency, and cause many more deaths, here. In fact, sometimes I laugh at myself and shake my head at what my U.S. colleagues would think, because compared to them, or for that matter, to my own habits when I worked in the U.S., I prescribe vastly more antibiotics. But I have seen that whereas in Wisconsin one out of a hundred children with a cough and a fever has a pneumonia, here eighty or ninety do. And untreated they die. Sometimes, even with antibiotics they die. And even among those of whom I say, oh, this time it really is only a cold, a very high proportion will return in a few days, and by then it will have become pneumonia.

As for me, fortunately I seem to be very healthy. I fall prey to an upper respiratory virus a couple of times a year (about the same frequency as in Wisconsin), often after an especially busy period in the life of the lodge or of the clinic. But, thanks to Explorama, I am well fed, and that, I believe, is the crucial edge that my patients lack. Every once in a while, though, I succumb to something else.

As I was on the verge of leaving Wisconsin to come here for the first time after my initial contact as a tourist, and was working frantically to wind up my Wisconsin practice, a fax arrived from Pam in Iquitos: "Study up on dengue fever," she warned, "there's an epidemic of it here in Iquitos." Dengue (pronounced DEN-gay) is an illness caused by a mosquito-borne virus of the family that includes yellow fever and St. Louis encephalitis. The family is widespread in all the tropics, worldwide, and there are several strains of the virus, the worst being the varieties that cause internal bleeding, with high mortality rates. Fortunately, the strain in Iquitos did not appear to be the hemorrhagic type. It was, however, a genuine epidemic, with many cases reported.

Dengue is also known as "breakbone fever." This is not because bones actually break (they don't), but because severe bone pain is a peculiar characteristic of the disease—as are high fever, headache, pain in the eyes, and general malaise. Being a viral illness, it has no medical cure. Victims rarely if ever die of the nonhemorrhagic types, but they definitely are aware of being victims.

After being here for two or three weeks, I accepted Pam's invitation to go into the city and accompany her and her children to the festival of San Juan. It was an adventure all around—simply being in a completely Spanish-speaking environment was a challenge, and the fiesta and its attendant rituals were a great deal of fun.

A week or so afterward, however, I had to conclude that I had been bitten by the wrong mosquito, almost certainly during the festival. There came a day when, although I don't usually suffer from headaches, I had a dull thudding in my occiput all day long. But, I told myself hopefully, the location was wrong for dengue, which should cause pain behind the eyes, not at the base of the skull.

The thudding, however, became slowly worse through the day, and was followed by a sleepless night with not only headache, but also fever and shaking chills. Furthermore, when I got up in the night to go to the bathroom, I had to ask myself how I could possibly have sprained both ankles without noticing it at the time. And just for good measure, some unseen, unheard, unfelt person managed to sneak in under my mosquito netting and pound a knitting needle through one, then the other, of my shoulders.

The next morning, my eyeballs ached. Yes, it was dengue.

It didn't take long to decide I didn't care much for this virus. Every step I took jarred every bone in my body. My sternum felt as though someone had taken it out, gone over it a few times with a rolling pin, and then replaced it, where it crumbled with every breath I took. Not only my ankles, but also my knees and hips, it turned out, were sprained. And my eyeballs had become a pair of spherical aches in a head that throbbed quietly all the time, but really became obnoxious if I had the audacity to lower it. Picking up a dropped item from the floor made me wince. Most significantly of all, I lost my taste for drinking coffee and developed an unaccountable craving for hot tea.

But I figured I'd been worse, and I'd get better. My room was close to the dining hall and its supply of water and juices. I hid in bed, stepped as little (and as lightly) as possible, and within a week I had perked up and gone back to coffee.

I concluded that, given a fortuitous constitution and a little luck, even blond-haired, blue-eyed *gringas* can survive the rigors of the jungle. And there is nothing like being sick oneself to give the doctor a little more sympathy with her patients.

# CHAPTER THIRTEEN

# More Learning

In order to maintain my medical license in Wisconsin, I must engage in what is called continuing medical education, or CME. This is available to physicians through a variety of avenues—conferences, mail-order study courses, computer programs, and others. Although it would not be necessary to keep my Wisconsin medical license active, I feel a little more secure by doing so; thus I subscribe to a number of journals and once every few years even make it to a conference.

The legal requirements, however, are not the only reason to try to maintain currency. There is always the sense that the world is fast leaving you behind. Medicine is a rapidly changing field, and keeping up isn't easy, even in the developed countries. Here, cut off as I am from a physician's usual contacts—other physicians, visiting drug reps, regular medical journals, even odds and ends of information gleaned from television news or mentioned by patients—I need to try a little harder just to keep from falling too far behind. Even worse, I find that here I have need of skills that are not normally even taught in medical schools.

Thus it was that I found myself in Iquitos, where the most obliging head of the laboratory at the Regional Hospital had agreed to let me work for a week in the lab. In my jungle clinic, I have few of the accoutrements of modern laboratories, but I do have my microscope and a few reagents for performing simple tests. I knew that in Iquitos they would be using the same reagents for the same simple tests, and I hoped to learn from the expertise of the laboratory technicians there.

I arrived on a Monday morning, and got off to a slow start. The hospital is a large, airy building with a good deal of decorative brick opening onto weedy courtyards and with many bare counters, empty drawers, and unfilled storage areas, as well as crowds of patients jammed into the waiting areas in front of the various clinics. I wandered to the lab by a back route through the maze of corridors and was interested to find the back hall of the laboratory awash in an inch or so of water and being diligently scrubbed. Oh good, I thought, they try to keep things clean. I wonder if this is the usual Monday procedure.

It wasn't. The city water supply is always a little dubious, and the entire hospital had been without water for the whole weekend. A faucet somewhere had been inadvertently left on, and by the time the staff came to work early Monday, a minor flood had occurred.

So the lady with the broom swept and swept, coaxing the water away, and someone came with a wrench and talked to the faucet, and at about 9:30, an hour-and-a-half later than the official opening time, work began.

No one really knew what to do with me. Who was this *gringa*, and what was she hanging around for? The head of the lab, who had given me permission to be there, had not shown up yet. Nonetheless, the usual Latin courtesy asserted itself, and I was made quickly welcome. I spent the first day in the hematology lab, where blood specimens are handled. The man working there did so without using rubber gloves, which would be unheard of in the U.S. On the other hand, in the U.S., every lab has boxes and boxes of gloves. He did not have any.

We began by sorting out the work orders and numbering the samples. He went to the bucket holding yesterday's slides, which were being washed by an assistant, and we picked out the ones with the fewest scratches. He set the slides out on a staining rack, dropped on the blood samples, and showed me how to stain the slides so that the blood cells could be identified under the microscope. In a modern laboratory, most of this process, from the staining to the reading of the slides, would be done by fancy machines, requiring the assistance of the technicians only to make the actual transfer of blood to slide. However, it was good practice for me, since my jungle office does not have the same machinery that the Regional Hospital does not have. While we waited for the slides to dry, he washed more of the glassware, most of which was the sort of item that would be disposable in the developed world.

To measure hematocrits, tiny tubes were filled with blood, again with ungloved hands, and plugged with clay taken from the back lot of the hospital. A centrifuge was pulled from a locked drawer, and the tubes were set in it to spin. (The process took five minutes; with the hand-operated centrifuge that I had out at Yanamono, it was necessary to turn the eggbeaterlike handle for fifteen minutes, steadily and smoothly, in order to settle the blood sufficiently for this simple measurement, so this centrifuge looked pretty fancy to me.) After we had removed the tubes and read and recorded the hematocrits, we moved on to another test, which involved removing the blood from the recycled antibiotic vials in which it had been collected. He did this by inserting a glass measuring tube called a "pipette" into each vial and sucking on the other end through a rubber tube attached to the pipette. This is called pipetting by mouth, and has long since been abandoned in the U.S. in favor of using rubber bulbs to provide the suction. Again, however, this piece of equipment was not available.

On my way out at the end of the morning (the laboratory, as well as most other services in the hospital including the telephones to the outside, works only until 1:00 P.M.). I was slightly startled to find a horse standing in the lobby at the rear of the hospital. There is no door there, just an open entrance area, and apparently the hospital gives permission for a few livestock to graze its back lot. This one had simply decided to take a look inside. I called the man with whom I had spent the morning, and he laughed and shooed the animal out.

I spent the following day in the laboratory where sputum specimens were examined for tuberculosis. The bacteria that cause TB travel by way of airborne mini-droplets and are remarkably tenacious, surviving on lab counters for months even after having been wiped up following a spill. The technician here dug up a mask for me, as protection against infection by the organisms that must have been rampant in the air of the small room; he worked without a mask himself, though, and had done so for years. I mentioned it, and he smiled and shrugged and said, "Better to work with gloves, too, no?—but there aren't any. We can hardly get soap to wash our hands."

The day after that, it was the malaria program. Again, the blood specimens were taken from patients without the luxury of using gloves. And the next day, I went to the room where a young woman works with stool specimens. She had ONE glove, which she wore on the hand actually handling the specimens and which she washed at the end of the day, to be reused when she returned.

When I left at the end of the week, somewhat wiser in the ways of the laboratory and much touched by the conditions under which these people were working, I resolved to bring gloves and microscope slides back to this laboratory whenever I had extras. I continue with that practice to this day, and the materials are invariably welcomed with huge smiles.

A year or two later, I returned to the Regional Hospital in order to practice tubal ligations under local anesthesia. It is a great idea, and a service much needed here, where women begin to bear children as early as thirteen years of age and continue to bear every year and a half to two years until they reach menopause. When I first came here, tubal ligation was offered by the government, but it was too costly for most of the river people to afford, around forty dollars in U.S. terms. Now it is being offered for free, and Dr. Mejia had come from Lima to train local docs in the procedure.

The women showed up at the family planning clinic in the Regional Hospital, where they were interviewed and admitted, having previously been given pre-op instructions: leave your jewelry at home, come with an empty stomach, don't bring your children along, and so on. We doctors performed a brief exam in the clinic, then met the women upstairs in the third-floor obstetrical suite, which has several delivery rooms and one operating theater. I went to the nurses' station and was handed a cloth-wrapped packet containing scrub clothes, booties to put over my shoes, cap and mask, all made of cotton. In the U.S., all but the scrub clothes would be of disposable paper. We performed from two to six surgeries each day, and used the same scrub suits and the same covering gowns for all that day's surgeries.

The first step in any surgical procedure is to "scrub up." This means washing one's hands and forearms thoroughly with an antiseptic solution. In the Regional Hospital, however, as in most of Iquitos, there was no water issuing from the faucets past the hour of about 7:00 A.M. (This is not the same as when there is no water at all. The city's water pumps just don't have the oomph to handle the daytime demands, therefore water never flows during the day; the households that have faucets turn them on at nine or ten o'clock at night and fill basins and tubs and buckets in order to have water for the next day's use. The Regional Hospital does the same.) A large sink had been filled during the night, and we dipped water out of that in order to scrub. It was not the most sterile way to do it, since we had to take turns touching an unsterile container to scoop up the water, but it was what we had to work with.

Entering the operating room, I found a space pretty much like those in the U.S., that is to say, a largish room with an operating table in the center, an operating light overhead, no windows, and, unlike in the U.S., no air-conditioning, with an outside temperature of ninety degrees. This later proved uncomfortable, given the cotton scrub suit, the surgical gown over it, the cap and mask and booties and rubber gloves. Each patient entered in turn, climbed onto the table, and was connected to the same liter of IV fluid, in order to deliver the drugs used for the anesthesia. In addition to the lidocaine that was injected at the site of the incision, we gave 10 mg. of Valium, a dose of a synthetic narcotic, and a touch of atropine, all by vein. Ketamine, an intravenous general anesthetic, was on hand, should any of the women need a little more calming down.

The needles plugged into the women's arms were disposable, and each woman came with her own, but one liter of fluid served for five or six women, and I am not at all sure that the tubing for the fluid was changed, either. The cloth covering the table was not changed between women unless it had become particularly gory or sweaty, and although we did change gloves between patients, we did not re-scrub. There was a clean instrument pack for each new patient, but the scalpel blades had clearly seen better days. And two days into the procedures, I realized that we were using the same syringe to inject the local anesthetic into all the women.

U.S. physicians, take note. The supervising surgeon was quite strict about not plumbing around in the abdomen any more than absolutely necessary, and made us use instruments instead of our gloved hands when we did have to reach inside. But the operating conditions were not as ideally sterile as they would have been in the U.S., and these women were given no antibiotics. Nonetheless, postoperative infections were almost unheard of. There was one, I believe, among a hundred or so patients.

We would never dare do things this way in a country where more sterile procedures are readily available, but it is heartening to know how much can be accomplished even when conditions are not what most Western surgeons would find acceptable. Furthermore, Dr. Mejia, who was clearly an excellent and most accomplished surgeon, was marvelously adaptable. The scissors isn't very sharp, he shrugged, but it's what we've got, so cut with it. His technique had obviously been learned in a fancier setting than the one we had in Iquitos, yet he remained even-tempered and patient throughout the whole time I worked with him, taking what was available and working with it, an attitude that I have found over and over among medical personnel in this area.

I have also had the good fortune to receive occasional visitors from the United States who brought their skills with them. One OB-Gyn, Dr. Gary Turner from Duluth, Minnesota, came and gamely helped to do a half-dozen tubal ligations in my own clinic. Our operating theater was a bit cooler than the one at the hospital since we have windows, and we had more drapes, running water, and supplies, but the conditions were nonetheless challenging, since we had little in the way of support staff. In the developed countries, physicians sometimes take their nursing staff for granted; in a place like this, where you must do for yourself what the nurse normally does for you, you come to realize just how important support staff personnel really are. Gary Turner began by asking for the ligation set, the group of instruments normally used for tubal ligations . . . but since neither I nor my two assistants, whom I had trained, had ever performed tubal ligations, there was no such set already gathered. Gary had to stop and think for a moment: OK, how many hemostats do I usually use? how many Babcock clamps? and so forth. He rose to the occasion, though, and most generously shared his skills with us.

At the same time, Dr. Maris Smalley, a Duluth dentist, visited, with his wife Fran to assist him. He brought along a portable head-rest that he clamped onto the back of one of our wooden chairs, fitted a piece of two-by-four under the front legs of the chair to tilt the seat back a bit, and bingo! we had ourselves a dental chair. He also brought dental explorers, elevators, extractors, mirrors—and plenty of dental needles and cartridges of anesthesia—and set up shop. He taught both me and my assistant to pull teeth, and carefully showed us how to clean and then sterilize the instruments afterward.

Dr. Bill Slack, an ophthalmologist, also loaned us his expertise. Pterygia are a very common problem here. These are overgrowths of the conjunctiva, the membrane that covers the eye. They are seen occasionally in the United States, usually among people who work outdoors, but are not very common. Here, though, it seems as though nearly half the population has them. When small, ptery-gia are simply heaped-up bunches of conjunctiva in the corner of the eye; but if unchecked, they grow until they cover the cornea, the clear window that lets light into the eye. Once the cornea is blocked, light cannot reach the retina, and the person loses vision. The problem is simple to correct. Under local anesthesia, the of-fending conjunctiva is scraped off the cornea and pushed back into its corner. The procedure takes no more than half an hour at most, and results in the restoration of sight. So Dr. Slack's personal course for us in how to perform this simple operation was yet another step toward better medical care in the jungle— even though, as with tu-bal ligations, cesarean sections, and pulling teeth, it was not a proce-dure that any internist in the United States would dream of doing.

Opportunities such as these are one of the rewards of this semi-wilderness practice: practitioners from other specialties freely and gladly share their expertise, enabling me to enjoy a far wider range of skills than I would ever be able to exercise in the ever more specialized United States. Of course, I'm not nearly as fluent at reading an electrocardiogram as I used to be, and a number of my other high-tech skills, such as inserting pulmonary artery catheters, are also failing. But I no longer live in that high-tech world, and for most of my patients, if I cannot do what they need done, they will not be able to get the help anywhere else. As far as I am concerned, the ability to be able to do minor procedures and lab work for my patients is a pretty good compensation for the loss of currency in the skills needed in that other, far away, and electrically powered world.

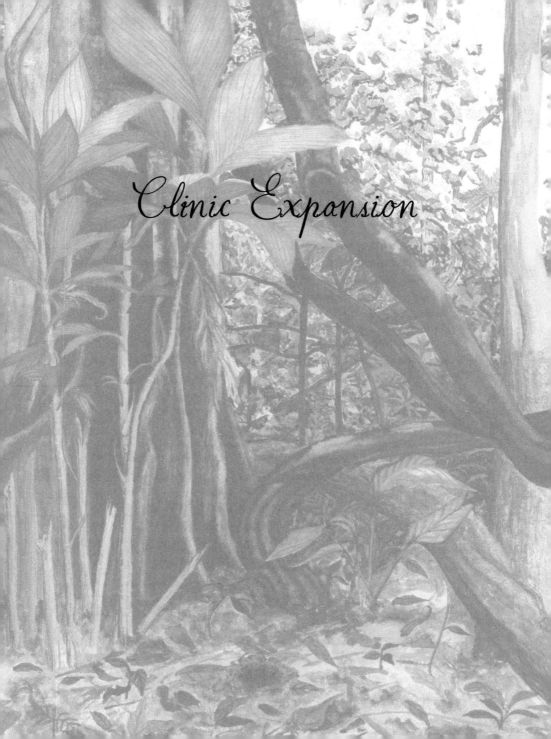

Clinic Expansion

CHAPTER FOURTEEN

# Rotary Rescue

After my first year and a half, the "clinic" was fairly well established and I was caring for about a hundred patients a month. At this point, the clinic contents still were limited to a few basic instruments, a bed doing duty as an exam table, and medicines stashed mostly in cardboard boxes, all located in one room with a kerosene lamp, a pitcher of water, and a thatched roof. I take a perverse enjoyment in "making do," but a real exam room, a second room for seriously ill patients, and more room for record keeping would have been most welcome. Sometimes, I even longed to be able to flip a switch and have the light come on.

I couldn't complain about the overall workload. Certainly, to a physician in the U.S., the total number of patients I was seeing would have amounted to a leisurely schedule, except for two factors: here, I had no help, and my patients came to the clinic in irregular patterns and at any hour of the day or night.

One hundred patients a month would be a halftime commitment, at most, back in my Wisconsin clinic. But in my Wisconsin clinic, where we were six doctors, we had a support staff of twenty, not even counting people like pharmacists and respiratory therapists available outside the clinic walls. When a baby peed on the floor here—and they do with some regularity, diapers not being a feature of life in this region—I had to stop and clean it up. I was keeping all the medical records, from writing to filing; instead of simply dictating notes to be typed by someone downstairs, I was writing the entire history, exam, and treatment plan by hand. I took all the temperatures and measured the blood pressures myself, chores that would have been performed by aides in Wisconsin. When medication was needed, there was no point in writing a prescription, since there are no pharmacies for miles; I had to hunt down the appropriate pills from my stock, count them out, search for a container, bottle them up, write the label, explain the directions carefully to my patient (especially for those unable to read), and then, if any money was due, collect and record that. I was also bookkeeper, public relations officer, community spokesman, quality control supervisor, and buyer of medicines and supplies. Of course, none of the daily work could even get underway until the floor had been swept and the plastic sheets had been pulled off the desk, the bed, and the bookcase where the medicines were stored. These sheets were necessary to protect everything from fallout from the thatch roof: dust, lizard droppings, bits of thatch, and the occasional more animate items. This fallout also made it necessary to dust and wipe things down frequently. These tasks, of course, fell into my job description as well.

Yet another problem had to do with scheduling—there was none. There were days when there were no patients at all (for instance, when I went into the city to purchase more medicines, or on holidays when would-be patients were too busy imbibing to take notice of illness), while on other days ten or twelve people would come at once, which under the working conditions constituted a challenge.

Worse yet, my patients had fallen into a jungle rhythm. No one would have expected a doctor in the city to attend them at 6:00 A.M.

But here, that was a very convenient hour—full daylight, everyone awake, still too early for breakfast to be cooked and too early to go to the fields. A perfect time to visit the doctor!

It would have been OK if I could have had an hour of peace before breakfast, done my laundry at midday, and rested at night; but the number of knocks on my door at odd hours was getting to be intolerable. It was astonishing how many people urgently needed for me to determine the nature of their rashes just as the late afternoon daylight was fading, making it necessary for me to peer at the lesions by the dim glow of lantern light. It furthermore began to appear that whole boatloads of people were carefully timing their arrival to coincide precisely with the sounding of the drums that announced meals at the lodge. On the day that I had sixteen patients, I decided that the time had come to proclaim clinic hours. Accordingly, I scrounged a scrap of plywood and a bit of leftover paint, and made a sign:

> La Clínica Yanamono
> Hours of Service
> 8:00–12:00 mornings
> 2:30–6:00 afternoons
> Sundays, mornings only
> Emergencies whenever

That last, of course, was a large loophole—anyone who is sick, with any ailment, at any time, feels that it is now an emergency: "Gee, doc, I stood it as long as I could before I came." People here are especially insistent on that point, and after all, even if it is just a cold (which I can't determine without doing the exam anyway) or a headache for the last twelve years, how can I say "come back tomorrow," knowing that coming entails four hours of paddling a dugout canoe?

But the "hours" did help. At least some. At least for a while.

Still, even with semiregular hours, there were limits, and I was approaching them. I was still a long way from burnout, but I like to look ahead, and when I did so I saw a steadily growing workload, with no end—or relief—in sight. I already knew that I needed help, and I also needed more room. I was going to have to find myself an assistant, preferably sooner rather than later.

As for more clinic space, I had no idea how I could even begin to meet that challenge.

Fortunately, I have periodic cravings for bacon, fresh asparagus, doughnuts, my family and friends, and the hills, trees, and rivers of Wisconsin. A trip home was in order.

While I was there, my longtime friend Dan Peterson convinced his office-neighbor, Jean Feraca, a formidable radio personality who airs two hour-long live interviews every weekday on Wisconsin Public Radio, that I should be one of her subjects.

After her interview and the call-in portion of the program had ended, as I was leaving the building, the office secretary told me there had been a couple of other callers who had indicated interest in my project and had left their phone numbers. The secretary offered me the use of her phone, so I could return the calls on the spot.

One caller was a man who expressed profound enthusiasm for a tree that grows in India and that evidently has the potential to pretty much save the world. Its roots stabilize the soil, its twigs make cavity-preventing toothbrushes, its leaves have antibiotic qualities, and I don't even remember what all else, but the list of its beneficial properties was lengthy and impressive. I wasn't completely clear as to what it was he was trying to say to me or why he was calling, but I believe that he was trying to convince me to carry a bunch of seeds to Peru and try to start a forest of these worldsaving trees there. I politely accepted his offer to send literature, but decided to hold off on the actual seeds. The other caller identified himself as an architect from Duluth, Minnesota, and a member of Rotary Club 25.

His club, he said, had built a dental clinic in the South Pacific, and he thought my work sounded like another potential project for them. What he did not say at the time, but that I realized later, was that he had been intrigued by his work on the dental clinic project; but, being a pure-blooded organizer and a persistent and determined fellow, what he really wanted was a project of his own to direct. His name was Jon Helstrom, and luckily for me, I was about to become that project.

My initial response was warm but not eager. It was clear that I needed more and better clinic space than what I then had, and I had hoped that sooner or later, someone, somehow would come along to help me do what I could not do alone. On the other hand, offers of moral support, empathy, good wishes, and even help had already been numerous, but so far none of them had actually materialized, so I was not about to leap feet first into confidence that this connection with Jon would be any different. Nevertheless, I gave him my parents' phone number in Kentucky, where I would be staying for the last part of the trip, and we parted cordially. I put him out of my mind and concentrated on bacon, asparagus, and riding the motorcycle.

To my surprise, while I was at my folks' house, a phone call came one night from a Jon Helstrom. Well, I thought, if he was going to be serious about this, I could certainly accommodate him, so we talked some more, he promised to stay in touch, and once I got back to Peru, a flurry of letters and faxes began to arrive from Duluth.

Seven and a half months later, I found myself at the Iquitos airport awaiting the arrival of the Saturday night flight, which was carrying two men whom I had never seen but whom I was nonetheless looking forward to meeting: Jon Helstrom and Joe Leek, an allegedly semiretired ENT physician from Duluth, whose jobs in the week they were to spend with me were to look at the lay of the land in general, the climate, available building materials, and other potential construction details (Jon), and to try to decide if what I was doing here was indeed worthy of an all-out effort on their part to help (Joe).

Never in my life had I been so excited at the prospect of meeting two men in whom I expected to have no romantic interest. Despite my never having laid eyes on either of them, they weren't hard to spot—two middle-aged *gringos* in sports jackets, near the head of the line of incoming travelers, looking eager and nodding firmly in my direction. (Jon grumbled later that I, to his disappointment, was not quite as advertised. I had instructed them to look for a tall, blond, gorgeous *gringa* jumping up and down excitedly, and he pointed out that my feet in fact never left the floor.)

They bounded out of the customs area with huge grins and firm handshakes for both me and the Iquitos Rotary Club president, who had been shanghaied into joining the reception party. Then they immediately started handing out candy to the kids hanging around. Jon is an archetypal Norwegian, medium height, with white-blond hair, piercing eyes set in a relaxed face, and a nonstop, perfectly dry sense of humor. Joe is tallish, lean, and balding, with the stern face and sharp questions of a surgeon, accustomed to moving right along, getting things done, and tolerating no obstacles. In the week they were here, they developed into good friends and invaluable clinic-boosters.

We went down to the lodge on Sunday morning, and the following day, a most fortuitous patient arrived. In fact, I couldn't have asked for a better illustration of the work I was attempting and the environment in which I was scrambling to provide health care. The patient was a woman with a "tumor" on her hip. It was about the size of a hen's egg. My off-the-cuff diagnosis was lipoma, which is a benign, fatty tumor, but Joe disagreed. Too hard, he pointed out crisply, and too irregular. "Besides, look at that fluctuant spot there— teratoma!" he proclaimed. We were, however, in agreement that whatever it was, she didn't need it, and it should be removed. (As it turned out, we were both wrong on the diagnosis. He was kind enough to take the whole thing back with him to Duluth, where the pathologists pronounced it a weird sort of calcification.)

I cut, Joe assisted and advised. "No, no, cut lower or you'll never get around it; use mattress sutures here, not simple ones, it's a high stress area." It was not an easy task—the mass was unwieldy, large, and liquefied in places, with a tail that ran down over the front curve of her hip bone. Joe had a grandstand view of my awkward working conditions. Since the bed had been designed at a convenient height for sleeping, not for operating, I had to half-kneel, half-stoop. Occasionally I straddled her in order to get at the tumor. And even with Joe aiming a flashlight into the cavity, the light from the curtained window was so dim that it was difficult to see well enough to do a good job. Of course, the operating conditions were the usual "clean, but not sterile." But we did it. And most importantly for the future of the clinic, the case was a perfect demonstration of what I was doing here, and how I was doing it. When we had finally finished, Joe left shaking his head and muttering things like, "Well! What a wimp this Linnea is. Complaining about conditions like these. You just can't satisfy some people. She should be sending aid to Duluth instead of the other way around . . . "—grandly facetious and clearly impressed.

I could tell I had found an ally.

Meanwhile, Jon was poking around, observing methods and materials of construction and making his own contributions to the growing body of evidence that this makeshift clinic needed their help. Just in case he missed the point, it was made for him when he came to the clinic one day and sat down on the edge of the bed, and before he could begin to speak, his perch collapsed under him. The termites had been at work on the wooden slats that supported the mattress.

In between watching me and a relatively voluminous flow of patients during the week, they walked in the forest, paddled a dugout canoe, and saw enough of the local life to give them an idea of what it was that had drawn me here. Before leaving, they promised immediate assistance in the form of a grant that I could use to provide for an assistant and to rent a couple more rooms from the Explorama Lodge for additional clinic space. They also promised to do their utmost to convince their fellow Rotarians back home to take on the project of building me a REAL clinic—although when they said it would take at least a year to organize such a project if, in fact, it were approved, they could not have missed the look of dismay on my face. I needed it now!

When they left, it was with warm feelings all around and with many assurances on their part that they would plead my case, and the case of the people living in the Yanamono region, to their Rotary Club colleagues back home. In the meantime, thanks to their generous interim grant, I now had the resources to find myself that much-needed assistant. I set out to do so at once.

CHAPTER FIFTEEN

# Juvencio

When people ask me how I discovered Juvencio, I am at a loss. How could I have known that he would turn out to be the invaluable resource that he has become? I can't answer that question very clearly, other than to credit my intuition and be thankful for my good fortune.

I did know him slightly before he came to work for me. His three small children were regular customers at the clinic—extremely regular. They all seemed to suffer from one diarrheal illness after another, until I finally convinced him and his wife to boil their drinking water. (The convincing took a bit of doing. If you consider how odd the water tastes when you visit a strange city, it isn't hard to imagine the vast difference in taste before and after boiling the muddy river water, and I suspect that acquired tastes in water are probably even more ingrained than tastes in food.) In addition to their frequent bouts with diarrhea, there were rashes and bronchitises and minor injuries. They seemed to be a mishap-prone bunch. I also knew Juvencio simply as one of the people who live around here, the way I vaguely know all the neighbors. He is a near-legendary soccer player, recipient of accolades even here, where the ordinary recreational soccer players demonstrate a level of skill comparable to that of most North American semi-pros. He seemed, as I saw him in passing, to be intelligent, honest, hard-working, and thoughtful.

One incident in particular stood out in my memory. In the early years, each time I returned to Wisconsin for a visit, people here found it difficult to believe that I would actually come back. They had never had a physician in the neighborhood, so why should they expect that one *gringa* would really come to stay? Although I did feel vaguely appreciated, in this culture people say very little about their feelings, and there were times when I wondered if anyone even noticed that I existed. But once, when I was about to leave for a month of ice cream and potato chips, Juvencio came to the clinic, alone. I asked him, "Yes? How can I help? Which of your kids is it this time?" And he answered that no one was ill. He had come solely to tell me that he and the rest of the community appreciated my presence here. He merely wanted me to know that.

I was impressed with his sensitivity, appreciation, and courtesy. Now that I had a chance to hire an assistant, he came immediately to mind. The only remaining questions were, would he faint at the sight of blood? and, if not, would he like to try working with me?

As luck would have it, he was delighted to have the opportunity. At that time, he happened to be employed, and his job was driving boats for Explorama. I checked with Peter Jenson first, to be sure I wasn't depriving him of a valuable employee. (I was pleased to find that Juvencio himself insisted on doing the same.) Peter, happily, gave his blessing. So Juvencio began to assist me. He started with the morning sweeping and cleanup routine, which in itself was a small but welcome relief. The Rotarians, besides providing funding for him, had arranged with Explorama to rent me three rooms in addition to the original one. Juvencio's initiation into the medical profession was therefore a massive cleanup and rearrangement of the clinic's newly expanded quarters. Not only was there the usual debris, but termites had launched a major takeover bid on the building in which the alleged clinic was housed. We spent three or four days sweeping, washing, dislodging the seemingly innumerable cockroaches who had taken up residence in the boxes where I was storing medicines, and rearranging everything in the newly allotted space.

Once things were in some vague semblance of order and word had got about that clinic was open again, patients began showing up. As they did so, Juvencio shadowed me. I walked him through each patient's history and examination, explaining what I was look-ing for and showing him the use of the stethoscope, ophthalmo-scope, blood-pressure cuff, and thermometer. Then I had him re-peat each exam as I coached him along. For each patient, we dis-cussed the various possible causes of the illness, and I tried to teach him how to narrow those possibilities down to one most likely di-agnosis. Then we went over the plan of treatment, taking into ac-count the apparent illness, the patient's age, weight, and condition (pregnant? malnourished? dehydrated?), and any other relevant fac-tors. On quiet afternoons, I would try to teach him a bit of anatomy, a bit of pathophysiology (the whys and wherefores of disease), by means of whatever I could illustrate with one of my small store of books or by a patient we had just seen. From the kitchen, I ob-tained a piece of fish skin, I gave it to Juvencio with a needle and suture material, and he practiced putting in stitches. I submitted to being pricked in the hand and the arm as he learned how to start an intravenous line, and I taught him how to adjust the mirror on the microscope to catch the most light. He learned with amazing facil-ity, hindered only by his perfectionism, which sometimes caused him to give up because he couldn't perform a task as well as he wanted to.

One day, as he was writing up a medical record for a patient he had attended a bit earlier, he apologized for being so slow. I reassured him that I thought he was doing just fine, but he insisted, no, he was way, way too slow. I tried to argue that I had no complaint with his progress, but he went on to remind me that his formal education had extended only through the six grades of primary school, in the one-room, libraryless school down by the river. Since that time, ten years earlier, he had written virtually nothing except, in the rare intervals when he was employed, his signature on paychecks.

I thought about it. Here was someone who wrote no letters to his family (they were all at his side, and anyway there is no postal service in the rain forest), no reports at work, no notes to be left on the refrigerator (no refrigerator, and no grocery list in any case). He didn't even write checks to pay bills. Since the age of twelve, he had literally had no practice whatsoever in writing. The realization made his progress even more remarkable.

Now, several years later, he is capable of examining a patient and reaching a diagnosis (the first and most important step—it is difficult to treat if you haven't decided what ailment it is that you're addressing), prescribing and administering an appropriate medicine, whether oral, intramuscular or even intravenous, and explaining the necessary follow-up for 80 to 90 percent of the cases we see each day.

However, there are certain inevitable limitations to his training. He will never know the more esoteric diseases, nor much about laboratory studies, since he has no opportunity to see these aspects of medicine. He will never know the difference, say, between rheumatoid arthritis and osteoarthritis. We don't see many neurological illnesses, hence he is not well-grounded in them. And, given the extreme shyness manifested by women in this culture regarding their nether parts (and his own reluctance to look; father of three, he attended not one of their births), gynecological experience has been difficult for him to obtain. He has, however, now delivered a baby on his own. And he can diagnose and treat conjunctivitis (pinkeye, in lay terms), sinusitis, external and middle ear infections, the common cold, pharyngitis, tonsillitis, bronchitis, pneumonia, asthma, the various types of diarrhea that we see (including cholera, which can be life-threatening and which often, by the time it reaches us, requires intravenous rehydration), skin infections both bacterial and fungal, abscesses, adenitis, and minor trauma. He may not know one type of arthritis from another, but he does know how to treat arthritic symptoms and can work out the complicated dosage schedule for a course of steroids. He can put in sutures. (That fish turned out to be a pretty good teacher.) He knows sterile technique and is a very capable assistant when I do anything surgical, such as the occasional cesarean sections we perform. He can himself incise and drain an abscess, tape an ankle, put on a splint, administer snake antivenin, and deal with allergic reactions. In my absence, he routinely handles life-threatening illnesses very capably (although not without a few qualms). He has also learned to pull teeth, and with his greater forearm strength does a better job at that than I do. Someday, when we have a drill, he'll do fillings, too.

And, of course, he can perform minor electrical and plumbing repairs, wield a saw, carve a graceful paddle for a dugout canoe, throw a cast net, and play a more than respectable game of soccer.

Although he has become virtually indispensable to me, his position does cause him a few problems. He sometimes suffers from the prophet-in-his-own-land syndrome—there are those who have known him for years and are skeptical that he can really do anything medical. Play soccer, sure; treat an illness—come on. But people who come from farther away and know him only in his professional role trust him more readily, and even among the locals, his reputation is slowly growing.

Then, too, he is very clinic-dependent. I sometimes wonder if I haven't created a situation he will some day come to regret. If I were to die tomorrow, or otherwise move on, he'd be out on a fairly slender limb, unable to transfer his hard-won abilities to any other setting, since despite his considerable skills, he holds no degree, no title, and no certificate attesting to these skills. This is doubly a shame, since his expertise far exceeds that of many nurses and approaches the level of at least some of the doctors in this area. His abilities, and his function in the clinic, are those of a physician's assistant. But in a country hopelessly enamored of documents, seals, signatures, stamps, titles, red tape, pomp, and ceremony, the absence of a degree is conspicuous and occasionally chafes noticeably on him. I would like to wrangle some sort of equivalency degree for him—but difficult as that would be in the U.S., it will be much more complicated here, owing to the aforementioned dependence on tape of a scarlet hue.

Nor is it likely that he will ever have the opportunity to receive more formal education. Even if someone would come up with the money to support him and his family for the years it would take, he would first have to complete secondary school (five years), then pass the admission test for medical school, competing against those with the wealth to have been sent for all of their educational lives to private schools, and then hang in through seven years of university-medical training, plus his postgraduate years. Even nursing school would require those five years of secondary schooling first.

But if he stays with the clinic (sounds good to me, I have come to rely heavily on him), he will continue to learn and grow in both ability and responsibility; and I hope that one day, when I grow old and/or tired, he will be able to carry on.

My hope is to continue this process. Juvencio was the first to come along, and has received by far the most intensive education. Despite the limits of my knowledge and the inevitable gaps caused by his lack of background in such subjects as chemistry and by the paucity of books and teaching aids, he has been a brilliant student. His successors regrettably receive less of my attention and time, as we are now simply busier with day-to-day clinic work, and I more often have to say, "Here, I'll do it so that it gets done quickly," which obviously is not the best way to teach.

Still, we try. The next generation of clinic aides is coming along nicely, in the form and face of Edemita, Juvencio's older half-sister. We have also had a few students from the nursing school upriver in Indiana. They come for three months to do their practical studies, and I anticipate there will be more of them in the years to come. These young people also represent a potential source of future clinic workers, although they're pretty green when turned out of the school—they have had no experience with any sort of actual patient care whatsoever, and cannot even take a blood pressure or read a thermometer when they first arrive. And I angle for a newly hatched Peruvian doc to be "on staff" here. One day, I will succeed in capturing one of these fellows; then the clinic will enter a whole new area of involvement in the training of local medical personnel, and Juvencio and his successors will have the benefit of another viewpoint (besides mine) on the practice of medicine. But with or without other clinic personnel, I have one superlative assistant in the person of Juvencio Nuñez Pano, and remain grateful to him for all the hours of work that he has saved me and all the times that he has pointed out something that I might otherwise have overlooked.

At the time his career was launched, however, when my sanity was at least temporarily saved by that generous interim grant from the Rotary Club of Duluth, the "real clinic" had yet to materialize. Having solved the immediate problem of finding my assistant, I turned my energies toward awaiting word on the fate of Jon Helstrom and Joe Leek's proposal to their Rotary fellows back home...

# CHAPTER SIXTEEN

# Building the Clinic

After Joe and Jon returned to Duluth, several months of ever-more-intense correspondence followed, involving questions and answers and research on my end and the same on theirs. For starters, if the rest of their Rotary colleagues agreed to this project, a site would have to be found, and permission obtained to use it. Although I tried not to get my hopes up, in case the project was rejected by the larger group, it was next to impossible for me to keep that resolve.

So, I waited. We exchanged more faxes. I waited some more. Finally one afternoon I was called to the radio. It was Pam, calling from Iquitos to tell me that she had received a fax announcing that the clinic would indeed be built. I let out a whoop that must have been heard in Duluth, and raced down from the radio hill to give a startled Juvencio a twirling, dancing, bearlike hug that lifted him off the ground.

In January of 1993, Jon returned, this time in the company of Bruce Von Riedel, a fellow Rotarian and building contractor from Duluth. I spent this time in deep consultation with Jon; he, as the architect, attempted to ascertain from me, the layperson, just what it was that I really did want in my soon-to-be clinic.

Jon ultimately came up with a plan for a clinic thirty feet wide by sixty feet long, to be built on stilts to avoid the annual floods but otherwise of North American-style construction, with solar panels to provide electricity and with a well to provide water. The plan showed a large waiting area in front, an office, a pharmacy, a room for overnight patients that would easily hold three beds, a small kitchen, a small laboratory, two exam rooms, a shower, a flush toilet, two "call rooms," (the quarters where Juvencio and I would stay in the event of a patient who required overnight care, since the site available to us was on the banks of the Amazon, a good fifteen minutes' walk from the lodge), and a laundry room. There was even a plan to build a small house for me close to the lodge, where I would continue to eat and socialize.

Wow.

Jon didn't unveil the complete plan until the night before he left, which meant that I got the job of coordinating a bewildering array of building supplies.

Purchasing lumber here, to give just one instance, is not quite as simple as it is in the U.S. You don't just go to the lumberyard and place an order. Here, you go first to the sawmill. The sawmills are located in the port area, where the road ends and you wade through the mud churned up by the huge trucks, to arrive at a small cabin where a secretary sits. You determine from this person if the type and quantity of lumber you require actually is, or soon will be, available, and arrange for it to be cut. The tree trunks are then removed from the waiting barges and cut to the desired dimensions. It is a good idea to be there yourself to assure that not too many wiggly pieces are included with the lot. Then you hire day laborers to carry the freshly cut lumber through the mud and up to where your trucks wait to take it to the warehouse you have rented, and there you hire another group of laborers to unload it and set it up to dry for six weeks, under the eye of the watchman you have hired to keep the lumber from disappearing. Once the wood is dry, you return with yet another group of workers, load everything again onto a truck, and take it to the finishing mill where the (extremely) rough-dimension lumber is planed, tongue-and-grooved, and so on. Then it is back to the warehouse, to wait until it is time to load again, this time onto the trucks that will take everything to the port, where it will be stacked on the barge that will deliver it to Yanamono, fifty miles downriver.

All this was especially tricky since, being go-ahead kind of guys, Jon and Bruce had arranged for the building crew to arrive within a month and a half of their visit here.

Fortunately, the work didn't fall entirely on my shoulders. Contact had been made with the Rotary Club of Iquitos, one of whose members was a carpenter-turned-builder, whose brother owned one of the few mills in Iquitos capable of producing the tongue-and-groove edging that Jon wanted for floor and ceiling boards. The Iquitos Rotary also generously volunteered to rent a barge to transport the entire load downriver. Meanwhile, the Rotarians back in Duluth and Thunder Bay, Ontario, Canada, egged on constantly by Jon, had gone about the complicated business of raising about $35,000 to purchase the lumber, the tin roofing, the hardware, the solar panels, the batteries to store the solar energy, the light bulbs and wiring, and all the miscellaneous other materials that the project would require, as well as to cover the cost of digging the well.

All that was left for me to do was to dash into Iquitos every time a fax arrived from Duluth with a change to be made or a question to be asked; to arrange the purchase and transport of nonlumber items like roofing, plumbing supplies, water tank, hardware, and wiring; to organize the work crew at this end to plant the support pilings; to clear a space where my house would be built; to order the necessary jungle woods (such as the heartwood support posts and the ridgepoles, rafters, and roofing for my house) to locate and negotiate with the well driller; to secure the agreement of our landlord-to-be; and, of course, to continue running the clinic.

The last week before the arrival of the construction party was a maelstrom of activity. I went into Iquitos in midweek, as the barge, and delivery of all the building materials, had been promised for Wednesday. Wednesday, there was no barge. But Thursday, there would be. Thursday, there was no barge. But Friday, *sin falta* (without fail) there would be.

By Saturday morning, I was getting nervous. Thirty-five North American Rotarians from Duluth and Thunder Bay, all eager to begin toiling under the unrelenting tropical sun, were due Saturday. They were to boat down to the lodge the next morning and were expecting to commence work Monday. What if there were nothing to work with?! But progress was finally being made. By Saturday morning, a crew of what appeared to be soldiers (in Iquitos, it pays to know the right people) were busy shuttling the mountains of wood onto waiting trucks. The builder took me to the port, and at that end, the wood was forming a growing mound on a barge that could have carried half the rain forest in one trip (and probably did, for most days of its working life).

It looked promising.

The plane came in on schedule despite a blinding rain, and disgorged a crowd of beaming Minnesotans and Canadians. All were met by the president and other highly placed members of the Iquitos Rotary Club, along with their wives, and bouquets of fresh flowers were presented to all the incoming Rotary females—a very gracious touch, and one that I had not anticipated. Greetings, salutations, and good wishes were exchanged and assurances were given that gasoline would be provided by the morning for the barge. The mountain of luggage and building supplies all made it, miraculously unscathed, through customs. Jon had brought a wooden crate filled with a hundred and twenty pounds of roofing nails and hardware; Roly, the plumber, had brought not only his plumbing tools and assorted pieces of tubes and pipes, but the kitchen sink, literally; and others were similarly encumbered. Finally, the new arrivals were taken to their hotel and tucked in for the night.

The following morning, we all went down to the lodge. I walked with everyone out to the building site to admire the forest of support pilings: seventy-two pillars, each six to eight inches in diameter, sprouting in orderly rows from the bare ground in the middle of the sugarcane field. Then I went racing around to all the local households I could reach, enlisting extra hands for the unloading process the following morning. This would ordinarily have been a simple task. But this happened to be the culmination of Carnaval, which here in Peru begins on New Year's Day and continues in an ever-upward spiral of revelry until it bursts to a spectacular finish at the end of the week that we in the north simply call Mardi Gras. Thus, the people I encountered that afternoon were all covered in mud, ashes, and paint (all part of the festivities) and tippling freely. It seemed likely that many of those with whom I spoke would be unable to get out of bed for the next three days.

The following morning, we all trooped out to the muddy building site, our work gloves on. The barge had finally arrived late the previous evening. To my delighted surprise, we were joined by thirty or forty of the local residents, from as far away as Yanamono upstream and Sapo Playa downstream. The crew even included a few of those whose sobriety had seemed so unlikely the day before. The pile of materials on the barge was immense: enough lumber for 1,800 square feet of floor, framing for interior and exterior walls, paneling for the ceiling, lumber for furniture and front and back stairways, doors milled in Iquitos, three hundred sheets of tin roofing, electrical wiring, a 150-gallon fiberglass water tank, solar panels, and several tons of other supplies.

A good-natured rivalry quickly developed, especially among the younger workers, to see who could carry the heaviest load. There was much muted surprise when the local folks saw the *gringa* women carrying and hauling side-by-side with the men (even though a few of their own women were doing the same). There was only one accident, when an overenthusiastic Rotarian stepped too close to a precarious pile of lumber and it toppled, scraping his shin rather badly. No broken bones, though, and no one got knocked in the head by the unwieldy fifteen-foot planks, no one fell off the barge, and I didn't even hear any complaints later of sore backs. The following morning, the Rotarians began what would become their pattern for the next three weeks: out to the sugarcane field by 6:00 A.M., carrying a giant thermos of coffee and a bag of rolls. Work until noon, break briefly for lunch, swear they were going to rest for a couple of hours until the worst heat of the day had passed, violate that oath and be back on the building site by 2:00 or so, and work until it got too dark to continue.

They did take it little bit easier on Sundays.

The clinic took form with wonderful speed. First, all the twenty-foot poles that Don Pablo, Juvencio, and a couple of others had so painstakingly erected were cut off to floor level. Next, the posts were all cut level with each other and a beam and joist frame was constructed. By midway through the first week, the hundreds of boards used to form the floor were all in place. There was much nodding of heads and murmuring as the sidewalk supervisors watched the North American women wielding hammers and saws. (Fortunately, few observers were on the scene when I, frustrated at being trapped at the old clinic by a steady stream of patients and determined to hammer at least a few nails in my own clinic, came out at the midday break and efficiently sawed off the floorboard on which I was leaning my weight, somersaulting through the joists to the ground below.) The four outer walls were built on the new floor as frames, each the length of one entire side of the clinic. As each was completed, the whole crew got together and hoisted in unison to raise the frame upright, where it was nailed in place by temporary supports, pending the application of the boards that would form the exterior walls.

The roof came next. There was a thirty-foot span from one side of the clinic to the other, and there were no thirty-foot beams. Bruce, the foreman, called a hasty consultation between himself and one or two others, and they came up with a design for a roof truss, which was then implemented, each truss finally being lifted into place by a complicated series of ropes and people.

Through all of this, Gene Cotton and Dave Rutford had set up what we soon were calling the furniture shop. Working on a hastily assembled floor and sheltered by a blue plastic tarp, they used drills and lathes and other fancy U.S. power tools they had brought from their own workshops at home, all powered by the three generators that they had also brought. They produced a seemingly endless array of chairs, benches, tables, beds, bookshelves, cupboards, and everything else they could think of that the clinic might need or want within its rapidly rising walls.

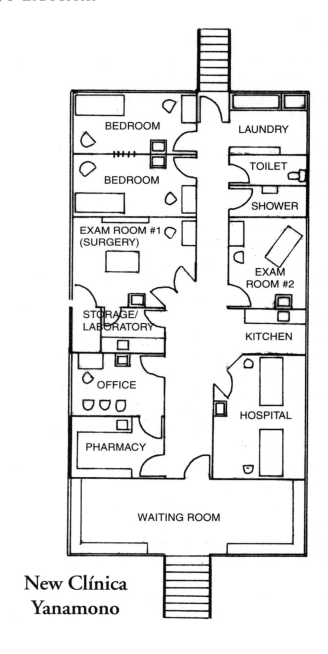

**New Clínica Yanamono**

On the third Sunday after beginning construction, the president of the Rotary district sponsoring the project arrived for a visit. Although the clinic was far from complete, by this time it did have exterior walls, interior walls, a roof, some furniture, and cupboards. On a Sunday afternoon, we festooned the yet-unscreened front windows with swags of gathered and twisted toilet paper, and held a dedication ceremony. To an audience of all of us *gringos*, a hundred or so of the local residents, and a visiting delegation of Iquitos Rotarians, thanks were expressed from all sides, and Jon presented me with the "key to the clinic," fashioned by the furniture makers out of yet another scrap of lumber. Then we all adjourned to the schoolhouse, where we were joined by another two hundred or so people; serenaded by the lodge musicians and emboldened by punch made of sugarcane rum mixed with milk, egg, vanilla, and coconut milk (and served out of barrels by our new landlord), we danced the afternoon away.

The work came to its eventual close just as the waters were rising seriously. As the main body of the crew left, three-and-a-half short weeks after arrival, the water was creeping out of the stream banks and over the paths we had been using each day. The Rotarians' last chore before departure was to load all the boxes and instruments and two recently acquired exam tables from what I was now calling "the old clinic" into open boats and then to haul it all down to its new home. By the time the water finally crested, the wisdom of building on support pilings would be amply demonstrated, as the clinic would be standing in three feet of water and we would be going to work each day in dugout canoes. The work still wasn't all finished, of course. My house lacked niceties such as doors, and the clinic itself was an unpainted shell. It took three days of sitting on the floor of the newly built pharmacy just to decide where to put each bottle of pills, and everything from exam tables to thermometers to cotton balls had to be assigned a place. The windows had no curtains, the well had not yet been dug (and when it was and we tried to connect the toilet, we found that the Peruvian version of that article was on the leaky side), the beds had no mattresses. Also, the weather had been rainy the whole time the construction was going on, so before painting could even begin, walls, cupboards, and ceilings as well as floors had to be cleared of the mud that had been tracked over the wood when that wood had (oh, so recently!) been lying at the edge of the cane field. It was during this phase that I came to a full realization of just how many square feet of surface there were in this immensely satisfying building, and I hardly knew whether to offer thanks or ask them to take the whole thing back, on grounds that it was just too much.

I opted, of course, for the former.

And the first time that I was called to the clinic at night for a sick baby and I walked in the front door, pulled a string, and light came on, I stared at it in amazement, and thought, this is like being God: Let there be light.

And there was.

Simultaneous with the clinic construction, the other, smaller project dear to my heart was also underway: my house. Explorama had always let me live in one of their rooms, and for the last year and a half, I had lived in a large, screened-in room at the far end of the older, seldom-used house. It was a great location, fairly isolated from tourists (so they didn't get woken up when I was called out at night), large enough to accommodate a hammock and a double bed, and I appreciated the screening.

The problem was that it was also the room used by the katydid hunters and other bug scientists (my walk-in closet had actually been built by the Smithsonian Institute's katydid experts as a cage for their insects), and every time they came to visit, I had to move out. Jon Helstrom and his crew had therefore agreed to build me a small house of my very own, located about three-minutes' walk from the lodge dining room, on a patch of land where the very first Explorama shelters had been built some thirty years earlier. The land had long since grown over, but it was cleared and footings were set for a house approximately twenty by twenty-five feet in size. Local labor had been used to build the house's frame and the thatch roof; then the construction gang of Rotarians came and leveled all the foundation footings and built a plank floor, a wall separating the front room from the back, and waist-high walls in the back room. Above those walls, and from roof to floor in the front room, they put screening. The front room is tool room, sunroom, and clothes-drying space. Its only furniture is a built-in toolbox, a wooden file cabinet, a tiny desk, a plastic lawn chair (for my guests, if any), and a chair I made out of two hunks of foam rubber. In the back room, I have my bed, a working desk, my foot-powered sewing machine, and a couple of shelf units that hold clothes and books and the other accumulated junk of living. As in the rest of the lodge, my light is a kerosene lantern, which perches on a little shelf of its own, and my water supply is a pitcher and bowl, which I fill from the shower located out the back door and fifty feet away. In the years when there is flooding, the house can stand in as much as three feet of water, and then I come and go by dugout canoe. It's a simple place to live, but adequate for my needs, and decorated and made classy by the antique brass doorknobs brought by my Wisconsin friends.

The Rotarians didn't stop there, either. At least a few of them were so enchanted that they dreamed up other projects for future trips. One crew came back in late 1993 and built the "hammock house." This is a separate structure, just one large room with a roof and a floor and walls on three sides, where patients and their families can camp out if there are no boats back to their villages for a day or two. Another group returned just to spiff up the electrical system and build much-needed shelving in the pharmacy, closets, and storage spaces of the clinic. And finally, in early 1995, the last phase of construction provided us with a four-room clinic addition out in back, which serves as housing for visiting students, "call room" for me to stay in when I am there at night (freeing up my original room to serve as dental clinic), extra storage, more bed space for use when our patient beds are filled, and whatever other uses we can think of. The entire assemblage, though simple by U.S. standards, constitutes a very complete and self-contained clinic. Visiting tourists often comment on how elegant it seems, given that it is situated in the midst of a sugarcane field, in a country not known for its rural health care facilities. For my part, every day when I see it, I admire the efficiency of its design, which allows us plenty of space in which to work and yet can be maintained by my small staff.

And whenever there is a quiet moment, I look around at my clinic, with two exam rooms, office, pharmacy, lab, overnight room for patients, laundry, dental room, shower, bathroom, student housing, and all the rest, and I wonder—how on earth did all this grow from one small armload of medical supplies brought to the jungle way back in June 1990 by one eccentric (even slightly loony) Wisconsin doctor looking to do something different?

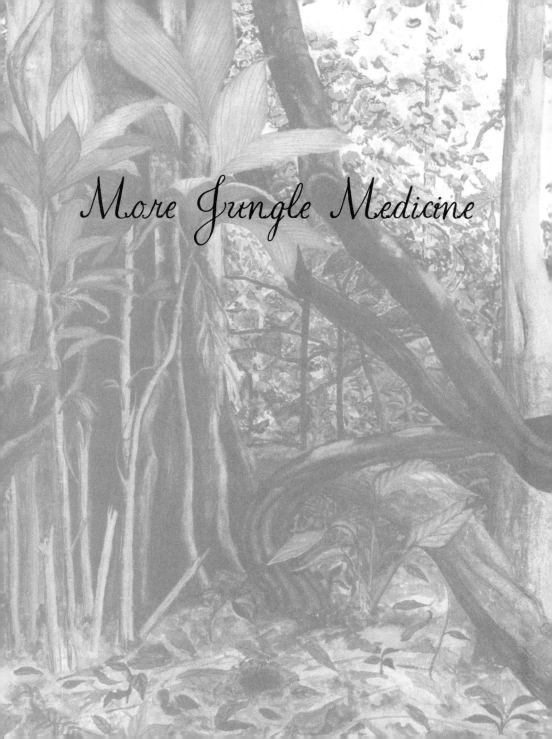

More Jungle Medicine

CHAPTER SEVENTEEN

# Trauma

Because the rain forest has no motor vehicles except for boats, and very little industrial machinery, our cases of trauma are few. Machete cuts are relatively frequent and occasionally serious; axes fall into the same category; people occasionally find a way to fall from the roof or from treetops. We also saw a five-year-old girl who was helping her family feed sugarcane into the press, which is like a wringer washer. She must have held on a little too long, because the machine pulled her hand cleanly off.

But generally trauma in the jungle is unusual, much to my relief. There are sometimes exceptions, however.

I had gone to bed early one night in an attempt to sleep off the last remnants of oroche fever (a lot like dengue fever, to which it's related, but with a dry cough and a runny nose thrown in for good measure). Around eleven o'clock, I awoke to the sound of footsteps approaching my room and then the inevitable soft voice at my door. The patient, as it happened, was Juvencio's father, Odorico, and the complaint, a gunshot wound to the foot. It seemed he had been out hunting, at night, in the forest, alone, and had tripped a gun trap set by someone else. Much of the hunting around here is still done by blowgun. More than once I've been startled, as I was walking along the paths, to find myself face-to-face with someone whose silent approach I had never heard and who held a nine-foot-long blowgun in his hand—but there are a few firearms. The type of trap that Odorico had tripped is technically illegal, precisely because of the danger of accidents such as the one that had just befallen him. They are tempting to use, however, because the owner can be in bed while his next day's dinner is hunting itself. The gun is simply propped on the ground, with a string running from its trigger to a trip wire across the path, in front of the barrel. The animal, or, occasionally human, who steps in front of the muzzle thereby initiates his own demise.

According to Juvencio, this particular trap had not been well set; if it had been made properly, the gun would have been aimed higher, in which case it would have done even more damage. As it was, the shell had ripped through the lower part of Odorico's heel.

To me, the wound didn't look too terrible—at least it wasn't in the abdomen, I kept reminding myself. But it was fairly impressive to the rest of the onlookers, who had all stayed, out of both spectator interest and the necessity to wield various flashlights to help illuminate our dim "operating theater."

The patient himself was wonderfully stoic. (These things can be a terrible thrash if the patient is screaming and moaning and wailing about dying the whole time one is attempting to work on him.) As an additional bonus, due to his disinclination toward shoes, the fleshy, callused pad on his heel was quite thick, and this had served him well.

I told Juvencio the dose to give of synthetic morphine, and had him put on a tourniquet and administer the painkiller. Ordinarily, I wouldn't ask him to work on a family member. Medics of any stripe do not normally attend their own families, for obvious reasons, but if other hands aren't available, then we can't always observe the proprieties. Besides, Juvencio had already been summoned by the others, and clearly did not wish to be relegated to a spectator role. Using semisterile technique and observed closely by a medium-size tarantula perched on the wall near my instruments, I cleaned inside the wound itself, using a twenty milliliter syringe to squirt saline through the injured area and knock the debris loose, and picked out small bits of leaves and trash with forceps. Two shotgun pellets washed out in the process; using a thin metal rod called a probe, I liberated two more. The prize, however, was the shell casing. When I spotted a hard white fragment, I just knew it had to be a chunk of heelbone. But when I was finally able to maneuver it into a position from which I could grasp it with the forceps, Juvencio said, "That's the *bala* (bullet)." As I tugged at it and very, very slowly was able to work it loose and haul it out, it became clear that it was neither pellet nor bone, but the plastic disc found at the base of the shotgun shell, complete with a reinforced upper disc, and, finally, most of the cylindrical casing, which had fractured in a rough spiral.

That was good for a few oohs and aahs among the admiring crowd. Once the casing was out, my syringe-pumped rinse water flowed freely through the tunnel left in the flesh and spurted vigorously out the other side; that made an impression, too, as did the in-one-side-out-the-other passage of my finger as I went exploring for more pellets. I could scarcely believe the man's luck, but it appeared that he had escaped with the heel bone intact.

Miraculous.

There wasn't much more to do, once I'd teased out all the pellets I could find. Wounds like this one are best left open—close them with sutures, and it is very possible that horrendous infections will develop inside. Better to leave it all open, protect it from flies and other invaders, and let the injured tissues grow back, gradually, by themselves. Left to itself, the human body is a pretty miraculous healing machine. He did well, in the long run. Despite the marginally sanitary conditions of his debridement, he developed no significant subsequent infection. He also suffered no deformity of the foot and no lasting limp, although he did come back a couple of times in the next few months to have me remove a few more pellets that had made their way to the surface.

There was an interesting footnote regarding the legal ramifications of the incident. Juvencio informed me, without rancor but with a certain grimness, that the young man who had set the ill-fated trap could go to prison (no small matter, here) for having made such a device. It had been decided not to press the matter, since it was clear to all involved that the young man had meant no harm. But he was to be responsible for all of Odorico's medical expenses resulting from the accident—total charges that first night amounted to the equivalent of nearly $6.00, with about twice that much accruing in subsequent checkups by house call and office visits to remove the additional offending pellets. In addition, during the victim's recuperation, the offender would be expected to do the daily work Odorico normally performed to support his family: cultivate their small field, fish and hunt, and so on. This would be a heavy chore for the young man, as he had a wife and four children of his own to maintain as well. It seemed to me to be a simple and efficient system. It was clear that he was responsible; therefore he had to assume the responsibility for the damage done. Neither court nor judge nor lawyer nor jury was needed to confirm that, nor did he try to contest it. No suits for punitive damages, either, and none for mental suffering on Odorico's (or his wife's) part. Jungle justice.

Another night, another call.

To take care of matters such as clinic maintenance and to have someone present at the clinic at all hours, there are three employees for whom the job designation is *huatchimán*. (This is pronounced "wot-chi-MON" and is adapted from English, where it would be spelled "watchman.") The *huatchimanes* are protective, both of the clinic building and of me.

Thus, they were quite apologetic when they notified me at around 10:30 one Saturday night that there was a patient that they didn't think could wait until morning. They were at pains to explain that the location of one of the victim's wounds was such that, here, it was considered very dangerous. They apologized several times, aware that my medical training was different from some of the ideas held here, but repeated that as far as they were concerned, one of the wounds was potentially lethal. The patient, they said, was a ten-year-old boy bitten by a caiman, one of the alligators that live in the isolated blackwater lakes, where many odd creatures grow undisturbed. I assured them that it was no bother; a person bitten by a caiman certainly warranted immediate attention. I pulled on some clothes, took my flashlight, and hiked down to the clinic, keeping more than my usual eye out for snakes and, this night, caimans.

"Bitten" turned out to be an understatement. The boy had been walking home at dusk with a companion after playing soccer, and had tripped over what he thought was a log. The supposed log had then reared up and tried to bite his leg off. When the boy fell, the caiman grabbed him around the chest, preparatory to dragging him back home to Mrs. Caiman, where he would drown the boy, then consume him at leisure. Fortunately, the child's fifteen-year-old companion grabbed back, and managed to drag him free of the animal's jaws, meanwhile screaming for help. The adults arrived too late to capture the caiman, but reported that he was six to seven meters in length, roughly twenty feet.

Luís, the victim, was a trooper. He remained remarkably calm, although I believe he was grateful for the ketamine with which I put him to sleep before patching him up. He had four wounds. A corner of skin about two by two inches had been ripped loose in his right groin. (Another inch and a half, and he'd have been out of the running in the procreation department, but luck was with him.) Further down, a hunk of skin and underlying padding had been torn out of his anterior thigh. Beneath the missing skin, the beast's teeth had ripped into the thigh muscle, but apparently had come away with little or no meat. The muscle was torn but most of it was there. On Luís's back, the skin was peeled away from his right shoulder blade, but the muscle below was intact and the flap of skin was still attached. The injury that worried me, however, was the same one that had so concerned the *huatchimanes*. This was a two-inch jagged tear or puncture over his lower right ribs, from which air issued in a bubbling hiss every time he breathed out and rushed in every time he drew another breath. This is what is called a "sucking chest wound" (for the way it sucks air in), or a "punctured lung." The problem with this sort of injury is that the lung collapses due to the air trapped between it and the chest wall. This can make breathing difficult, since even though there is air in the chest, it is outside rather than inside the lung, and it squashes the lung besides. I assured the *huatchimanes* that in my country, we, too, consider this to be a serious sort of wound.

However, young people often tolerate one collapsed lung pretty well, and Luís didn't seem to be having trouble breathing. I tried to insert a chest tube to serve as an exit for the trapped air. The tube didn't want to enter, so I inserted my finger instead, poking around hoping to discover an entrance. I found none. What I did find were the jagged ends of the rib that had been bitten through and that had punctured the lung (or perhaps the caiman's tooth had punctured it). Instead of the tube, I settled for a flutter valve, a loose floppy dressing sealed on three sides and open on the fourth. It works like a piece of Saran Wrap over your mouth—the air can be blown out, but when you inhale, the Saran Wrap/flutter valve gets sucked up tight and won't let air in. If the lung isn't too collapsed, and if some of the air that has already gotten into the chest sneaks out through the open side of the valve as the patient exhales, and if no more air is allowed to enter, sometimes a collapsed lung can be stabilized by a flutter valve. It was certainly worth a try. I spent the next hour or two doing a not-very-elegant job of sewing up what I could. It could be debated whether I should have sewn anything at all. Surgeons and emergency room physicians would have cleaned the wounds and left them open to heal by themselves, as I had done with Odorico's foot. On the other hand, in this climate and in the type of house where this child undoubtedly lived, flies are an ever-present menace, and leaving that much flesh open to the air seemed a worse risk than closing it. So I decontaminated everything as well as possible and sewed him back together as well as I could. I usually try to be neat when putting in stitches, but there was just too much work here to be able to linger over details, and the edges of all the wounds were torn, not cut cleanly. (I told him later that if he wanted pretty scars he should go for machete cuts instead of alligator surgery, but at least when he is older, he will have a great story with which to impress the girls.)

I saved the open chest wound for last, and when I got to it, the flutter valve seemed to have worked, so I closed him up tightly, in multiple layers to prevent further leaks.

When he came back the next week to get the stitches taken out, he was walking, although with a limp. His worst pain was not from the broken rib, but from the big open gash on his thigh, which was healing slowly.

And that is only one of several reasons why people around here are reluctant to venture out in the dark.

CHAPTER EIGHTEEN

# Childbirth

I've seen enough newborn babies to agree that some of them can be pretty cute. However, I've never felt particularly drawn to obstetrics.

Here, my distaste for obstetrics in general and jungle obstetrics in particular has increased for two key reasons:

1. If the delivery is normal, a woman doesn't really need the help of a doctor. After all, throughout history women have delivered babies without medical care. However, if the delivery is not normal, the complications can very quickly become life-threatening. I have neither the training nor the equipment and facilities to deal with such emergencies.

2. Babies really do prefer to come in the middle of the night—and usually the births to which I am called take almost all night. Since I practice alone I must stay with the mother for as long as it takes. Then, the next morning I must be prepared to see a whole clinic full of other patients who need me to be fresh and inspired and caring.

Despite my reluctance, however, babies insist upon being born, and they do not always agree to do so in the most straightforward and uncomplicated manner. Thus, like it or not, obstetrics is occasionally a part of my jungle practice. For example...

I had just sat down to dinner one night when Orlando, one of the room boys, came in to say I was needed "for a moment." Given the hour and the fact that people rarely venture out in darkness (because of the difficulties, and sometimes even dangers, of nighttime travel), I wondered if it wasn't just another joke, like the time they told me there was a patient and I looked all around the waiting area without finding anyone until I finally spotted the baby screech owl they'd captured. But he assured me there really was a patient this time, so I went. Out on the verandah stood Socorro, and the story she relayed was this:

Upriver a little way, Socorro had a niece, seventeen years old, who had had her first baby earlier in the day, around eight in the morning. She then proceeded to have a second baby, stillborn, three hours later. The placenta had followed, but she had lost quite a bit of blood; it was now twelve hours past the first delivery and the young mother was very thirsty and hungry but was throwing up everything she took in. And with each episode of retching she lost more blood vaginally.

I cursed my lack of obstetrical knowledge, but from the little I remembered from medical school it did not sound like a typical postpartum complication. It also did not sound like something I could assess, let alone treat, from a distance. Orlando armed himself with my large flashlight and we followed Socorro and her niece's husband down the rough track to the river. We motored cautiously upriver in a boat piled with damp and fishy-smelling nets, every now and again dodging floating debris or cutting the motor back to idle as we heard and felt a log bumping along underneath the boat. I brooded grimly over the paucity of my obstetrical knowledge and the possibility that not only might I be unable to help, I might not even be able to tell the family what was happening.

After twenty minutes we pulled over to a steep and slippery clay bank. At the top of the high bank was a narrow path between the cows and the cowpies, leading through a wooden gate and up to the plank steps of a fairly large house. Dogs barked and rushed out from beneath the house at our approach and were shushed and sent back by our escort.

We climbed the steps. "*Permiso* (May we enter)?" we politely asked, and "*pase* (pass)" came the reply. We entered a large open front room with forty or fifty people sitting or standing around the periphery, some talking quietly, a few playing cards, others sitting silently. This was the *velorio*, the vigil for the dead twin. We walked through, nodding to the assembly, and passed a small table on which lay the tiny stillborn infant, neatly swaddled, with a knitted cap on his head. His eyes were closed, and three candles burned around him. Later we heard the hammering and sawing as his miniature coffin was constructed. We passed through the doorway into the center of the house, where a wall of woven palm slats screened a mosquito net hung from the rafters. A knot of children followed curiously in our wake.

Inside, lying on a thin blanket on the floor, with a sheet of blue plastic beneath her to catch the blood, lay a young woman in the throes of what used to be called childbed fever. Her face and chest were beaded with sweat; although she was conscious and could answer questions once her attention was caught, she was distant and wanted to drift off into her own interior world. I had fortuitously picked up the thermometer in my hasty packing; it read 100.5 degrees, but she felt even warmer than that. I listened with my stethoscope, and her heart and lungs sounded normal, but she complained of pain when I pressed on her abdomen. Once I was able to get the crowd of onlookers to stop milling around on the floor that was creaking and groaning under their shifting weight, I could still barely hear her blood pressure at 70/50, with a weak and thready pulse of 130. A brief check (after I had shooed out the audience) revealed no obvious ongoing bleeding, and the uterus was firm, as it should be at this point, and not tender. The picture was one of infection and impending septic shock, which elated me. It would hardly have been appropriate to demonstrate my relief, of course, but relieved I certainly was. Inside, I exulted, "Septic shock! Infectious disease! Not an obstetrical problem, but a medical one. Something I can do something about!" I still didn't know why she should be so sick so quickly, but at least as an internist, I can deal with infection. We dug the IV fluid and the necessary paraphernalia out of my bag. I put a tourniquet on the patient's arm and was dismayed to find almost nothing for veins. I leaned over to check the other arm, narrowly missing the surviving twin as I crawled around in the confined space of the mosquito netting, but the other arm was even worse. Furthermore, the only needle I had with me was 20-gauge steel, an inch-and-a-quarter long—hardly a delicate or flexible tool with which to gain access to collapsing veins. My team of assistants (Pam, and Orlando's grandmother, who had attended the birth) moved the kerosene lamp a little closer and trained both flashlights on the girl's arm.

Fortunately, she was finally granted a little luck, and the huge needle slid into the vessel. Pam overcame her innate aversion to gore and held both the flashlight and the IV fluid until a string could be rigged from a rafter to hold the bag.

By the time the full liter was in, her blood pressure was up to 90/60, her pulse was stronger, her epigastric pain was less, and both she and I were breathing easier. She had not vomited in the time that we were there, her thirst had eased, and there was no more bleeding. The next step was antibiotics. In the U.S., these would have been intravenous, probably gentamicin and ampicillin; here we had to return to the Clínica Yanamono to retrieve the brand new, super-expensive cephalosporin so generously given to me by a drug rep back in Wisconsin. By the time we returned to the house, we found our patient already looking a bit improved. Her blood pressure was holding. Even better, someone had come by and left two vials of ampicillin. Since anyone can walk into any pharmacy in the city and buy any medicine they want, every community has at least a few vials of injectable antibiotics lying around in someone's house. Combined, these two vials would make up one adequate dose. I injected this, then got out the oral cephalosporin. I had already emphasized to the family the importance of boiling the drinking water instead of drinking it straight from the muddy river, as has been the custom here for centuries. Traditions die hard, though, not to mention slowly, and there was no boiled water on hand. So we waited, first for the water to be boiled, then for it to cool to drinking temperature. While we did so, I took the opportunity to look at our other patient.

The little fellow was red in the face, his skull was a bit uneven from his passage through the birth canal, and he was on the skinny side—not surprising for a twin; actually he was the larger of the two—but overall he appeared healthy. He was over twelve hours old by now; although not entirely forgotten, he was not expected to survive since it was believed that he would grieve over his dead twin until he joined him. Thus, no attempts had been made to suckle him. I offered him my little finger, and he clamped on it eagerly. I mentioned this, and a friend, neighbor, or cousin (I'm not sure which) who was currently lactating was summoned. When she arrived, she expertly and efficiently plied him with nipple until he finally caught on and nursed for all he was worth. I pronounced him handsome, and everyone laughed when I announced that I'd be back in seventeen or eighteen years to marry him.

Next, I crushed the tablet of Suprax, the expensive superdrug, and mixed it into a glass of the now-cooled water. The young mother drank it without throwing it right back up. When another fifteen minutes and a few more sips of water had passed without any vomiting, we began to pack up, leaving instructions for the remaining doses of antibiotics and promising to return in the morning.

For the fourth time that night, we traversed the darkened water, glowing under the canopy of stars, and the much darker footpath, arriving at the dining room of the lodge at just about midnight. On the trip home, I finally thought to ask when the young woman's amniotic sac had ruptured, and it turned out to have been four days earlier. Naturally, in all that time, she had been working daily in the fields and bathing nightly in the river. This solved the mystery of why she was infected—normally, a baby leaves the uterus shortly after the membranes break. After the first twenty-four hours, there is a dramatically increased risk of infection entering through the open cervix. After four days, it was no wonder she was ill.

The next morning, to my delight, both mother and baby appeared well. He had suckled again. She was alert and aware, if tired, had almost no fever, and looked well. Antibiotics really are miracle drugs. So we left instructions for giving the remainder of the antibiotics, along with strict admonitions to let me know if she did not continue to improve steadily, and departed for what I hoped would be the last time.

About the time I was wondering when the next obstetrics call would come, it did. This time the caller was Eduardo. He came by around 9:00 one night to mention that the newest baby was on the way and to get a bottle of iodine with which to clean the new arrival's cord. He returned sometime after 11:00 to say that the baby had changed its mind, and wasn't coming after all. Maria, he added, had now been in labor for twenty-four hours.

Eduardo is a small, slender young man with a delicately handsome face. His manner is usually a little hesitant, and his eyes hold a timidity that lives just this side of shame, or maybe fear. He apologized for the bother as we paddled across the stream in the dark and squished up the slippery bank and across the dark schoolyard.

Once at the house, Eduardo preceded me and worked his way between the mosquito net and the wall to crouch behind his wife, relieving the man who had taken his place while he had been summoning me. I felt sorry for him, as it did not seem to be a very well-organized birth. Usually there is an older woman who acts as midwife. There are also usually a couple of younger women—sisters or cousins or friends—fussing around, providing moral support, and helping with small chores.

But this time, beneath the mosquito net that crowded Maria right up to the wall, there were only the other two children and a toothless grandmother. Maria's contractions were strong and regular, her blood pressure was fine, and the baby's head was down far enough that it seemed he was probably past the narrowest straits. She looked tired of the whole thing, however, and was murmuring querulously about dying.

I reassured, and we waited. Eventually, the baby arrived, a little after midnight, making his birthday July 28th, Independence Day in Peru. When Eduardo called for someone to pass in the spool of thread with which he meant to tie off the umbilical cord, no one answered except, tearfully, his five-year-old daughter. Nor was there a *madrina* (godmother). The *madrina* or *padrino* (godfather) is the person who cuts the umbilical cord; conversely, whoever cuts the cord becomes the *madrina* or *padrino*. This role is taken quite seriously and entails a good deal of responsibility. The *madrina* and *padrino* really, truly are expected to be assistant parents, to take over if the natural parents should die, to be present at christening, baptism, school graduations, and other occasions of import, and to provide presents on all such occasions. If the designated godparent is not present at the birth, the baby remains attached to its placenta until he or she can be summoned.

In this instance, however, no *madrina* was in evidence. "Eduardo?" I asked. "Who is the *madrina*?—we need to cut this cord." "You can do it," he responded hopefully, but I shook my head. No, I explained firmly. I could not possibly be *madrina* to every baby whose arrival I attend. I could cut the cord, I offered, but as a physician only, not as *madrina*. I offered him the chance to do it himself, but he, in turn, declined. I cut the cord, and the child was *madrina*-less.

This home was truly a meager household, even by local standards. It was not the lack of physical possessions that made it so, but the utter lack of extended family, which normally provides wealth of a different sort. While in the United States the nuclear family is the norm, here an extended family is found under nearly every roof. In this home there were no grandparents, no aunts or uncles, no cousins, no social support of any kind—only two parents who were hardly adults themselves caring for an ever-growing brood of underfed children. This child, his siblings, and the two who were later to follow, were one of the strongest arguments for family planning.

Aside from my clearly well-founded distaste for obstetrics in general, and for jungle-style obstetrics in particular, one additional observation gnaws at me.

Not all these events are exactly joyous. The arrival of the sixth or eighth or tenth child in a family is often greeted with more tired resignation than eager anticipation. It is sad to see the plight of the families burdened with too many children, for whom there can never be enough food, never enough clothing, never enough opportunity for education, and sometimes not even enough love. Many times, the children of these families will perpetuate the cycle, caught in the bog of poverty. Sometimes I can't help but wonder what good it does to save the life of a child with pneumonia, if it only means that ten years from now, his own children will be dying from the complications of malnutrition?

Fortunately, the government of Peru, despite the country's being nominally 80-percent Catholic, has established a family planning program, in which they try, sometimes successfully, to provide free birth control supplies. There are problems, of course—women who stop taking their birth control pills during their menses or while their husbands are away; months on end when the program itself has no materials and supplies to distribute; women who cannot meet their appointment on the date prescribed because there is no canoe available; and distrust of a government that has too often in the past offered promises that it could not fulfill.

But progress is being made. Juvencio's sister Edemita, herself a grandmother since the age of thirty, practically grabbed the family planning program from my hands in her eagerness to promulgate it. And we are reaching more and more women like the one who has had twenty-four pregnancies in her forty-two years. Of these, she has carried twenty to term, and of these, eight—yes, eight—have died, leaving her with twelve living children (and I am afraid to ask how many grandchildren). She still has a few reproductive years to go, but has now chosen to participate in the birth control program.

One sixty-five-year-old woman came into the clinic one day with her ten-year-old daughter. Another mother-and-daughter team came together for family planning. This mother, at age thirty-six, had thirteen pregnancies, eleven deliveries, and six living children to her credit; the eighteen-year-old daughter had a one-year-old, a two-year-old, and a four-year-old. Still another mother in her mid-thirties, when questioned as to the ages at which three of her children had died, related how her daughter had died in childbirth at the age of fifteen.

Birth control is important everywhere in the world. However, to me it seems especially important here, where childbearing begins so early, where poverty is endemic, where the fish in the river are diminishing in both quantity and size, where the forest is shrinking, and where the possibilities for breaking the cycle are few.

So, in the clinic, I emphasize family planning as much as possible, as does Edemita, whose advice is far more valuable than mine, since it comes from someone who was raised in this culture and is far better able to communicate with the women we are seeing. Meanwhile, reluctant though I may be, I attend the childbirths that present themselves with as much grace as I can muster.

And I must admit that, once it is all over, sometimes it has been kind of fun.

CHAPTER NINETEEN

# Snakebites

My very first patient in the Amazon, way back when I was still a tourist, was a snakebite victim. Around here people walk barefoot most of the time, work in the cane fields, and bathe in the river. Since snakes of various types, many of them poisonous, thrive in this part of the world, close encounters between two-footed and no-footed denizens are inevitable. The meetings are more frequent when the water rises and the available dry land shrinks, forcing us all, snakes and people, into ever smaller spaces. Most bites are attributable to various species of *Bothrops*, of which the best known is the fer-de-lance. These reptiles are not as rapidly fatal as the mambas of Africa or the kraits of India, but they still cause about a 20-percent mortality. In statistical terms, this rate is substantial—especially if you are the victim.

Not only are the bites painful, terrifying, and sometimes fatal, but a myriad of beliefs and legends further complicate the issue. Prohibitions—against eating certain foods following a snakebite or having sexual contact while recovering from a snakebite—are widespread in the culture. I will probably never be familiar with all the injunctions. Sometimes questions even arise concerning the true identity of the alleged snake. Was it a snake at all, or actually a *brujo* in disguise? The answer obviously affects the approach to treatment. After a woman at Indiana was bitten by a poisonous snake, her family spent several days treating her for witchcraft before changing strategies and bringing her to the medical center. They arrived too late, for she died there of tetanus. Even if victims arrive promptly and have not been compromised by home remedies (such as concoctions that rely heavily on the power of sugarcane rum), there are still significant risks.

Antivenin, the first line of medical treatment, may itself provoke a potentially fatal reaction. On the other hand, there may be no antivenin available in the vicinity. Medical experts in the U.S. recommend administering, for starters, a minimum of four to seven vials of antivenin, and more later if necessary. My clinic rarely has that quantity on hand because the U.S.-produced antivenin is not to be found anywhere in Iquitos. One company in Brazil produces a perfectly good antivenin, but unfortunately that product must be smuggled into the country, so for obvious reasons there are occasional shortages.

One of the most grim cases showed up at my door on New Year's Day, 1995. A boat arrived on that rainy evening, bearing a pregnant nineteen-year-old mother of two. A snake had bitten her two days earlier, and she was being treated by the local herbalist. It appeared that the mode of treatment had been application of the "black stone." This remedy consists of a piece of charred bone, thought to draw the poison from the wound, held in place with a bandage.

Two developments had prompted her family to abandon the stone and decide to seek other methods of treatment. First, a neighboring villager had been bitten by a different but equally poisonous snake at about the same time as this patient and was also treated with the black stone. That man had just died. The second reason for the shift from traditional to modern medicine was that the woman had begun to hemorrhage. Bleeding signified not only that her own life was in danger, since she might bleed until there was no more blood left to lose, but also that she might lose the child she was carrying. When I first saw her at 8:30 P.M., the patient had no fever, her blood pressure was 120/80, her pulse was 64 and regular, and she appeared awake and in no acute distress. I saw no petechiae (pinpoint-size red bruises that signify the blood is not clotting adequately) in the membranes of her eyes. One lone petechia appeared in the roof of her mouth, but her gums were not bleeding. Her heart and lungs sounded normal and clear. Her abdomen was soft, with normal sounds, meaning that the intestines were still functioning, gurgling along as they should. A couple of small bruises on her hip showed where shots had been administered: one for pain, and one "to make the blood coagulate." The bite itself was just above her right ankle, near the Achilles tendon. Except for a couple of small cuts where an attempt had been made to suck out the venom, it did not look either severely swollen, blackened, or full of pus. Her foot hurt, but not too badly.

So far, so good.

The pelvic exam revealed that her underwear was clean, not bloody. The vagina showed no signs of recent hemorrhage. An examination revealed a closed cervix, so she did not look to be in imminent danger of losing the baby. I switched my headlamp off and shrugged my shoulders. No sign of hemorrhage that I could see, I explained to the family. Then the young woman indicated a need to urinate. We brought her a bedpan, and her urine came out bright red. Oh.

We gave her an ampule of antivenin. I also administered the antibiotics that I routinely use for snakebite, on the grounds that almost no one here is adequately vaccinated against tetanus. Snakebites usually occur on hands or feet that are caked with mud at the time of the bite and often inadequately cleaned thereafter. This certainly raises the risk of tetanus. I would be doubly grieved to lose a patient to that disease when the original problem was, after all, a snakebite.

Then we tucked her in for the night, and waited. In the morning she complained of abdominal pain, and her family reported that her urine looked the same as the night before. Her blood pressure was 104/66, her temperature and her pulse were unchanged. Her hemoglobin measured nearly normal. We put a sample of her urine in the hand-operated centrifuge and Juvencio cranked furiously for a few minutes. The results were alarming: her urine was 25% blood. That meant that the woman had nearly as high a concentration of blood in her urine as in her bloodstream itself. This was not looking good.

We gave another ampule of antivenin.

The following morning, she fainted while walking to the latrine. By this time, she had a fever as well. Her blood pressure still held steady, but her pulse was up to 100—a sign of either fever or blood loss—and her face looked pale. Her exam continued to be, in medicalese, unremarkable. The bite site itself was looking better. Her gums were not bleeding. Her heart and lungs remained clear. I could see no evidence of a miscarriage. She continued to have normal bowel sounds. But her belly had also begun to hurt, and by now her urine was settling out at seventy-five percent blood, with small ragged pieces that were probably shreds of bladder wall. We gave yet another ampoule of antivenin, along with a shot of vitamin K, which will reverse some types of coagulation problems. It usually has no effect in snakebite victims, but it couldn't hurt.

By mid-afternoon her urine was unchanged, she was even more pale and weary, and there was no indication that her downward slide was going to reverse itself. Her family wanted to return with her to their home. I couldn't argue with their plan since I had nothing else left to offer.

We never did hear of her outcome—one of the frustrations of working here is that you frequently lose track of your patients and never know whether or not your ministrations helped—but I am certain that she died.

In another instance of belated treatment, one forty-eight-year old woman was brought to the clinic three days after a bite by a *cascavel*, or rattlesnake. Despite their small size, these snakes are greatly feared by the people here. Their bites are quite lethal. This woman had been treated with herbal remedies and one shot of penicillin, since the family lived several hours away on the Napo River.

Unfortunately, by the time she came to the clinic, she was beyond saving. She had a fever of nearly 105 degrees and a pulse of 140, and her pupils did not respond to light. She alternated between breathing very deeply and rapidly, and breathing hardly at all—a condition signaling damage deep within the brain. Her hemoglobin was only 6.5, half of a normal level. My repeated calls could not get her to open her eyes, and she seemed oblivious to pinpricks on her arms and legs. She did moan and resist weakly when I lifted her left arm, however, probably because it was hugely swollen. Her hand, where she had been bitten, was black, and the skin had begun to pop open in small blisters. I immediately administered a vial of antivenin and some heavy-duty antibiotics, but sadly, she died about an hour after arrival without regaining consciousness.

The usual ways to die from snakebites in this region are by bleeding or through infection. Those who die of infection may succumb to tetanus or other bacterial contamination that was injected along with the venom or from gangrene that supervenes in the injured area when the limb becomes so swollen that blood circulation is impaired. Those who bleed may simply bleed to death or, if the bleeding is internal, may die from damage to the internal organs. The *cascavel* patient, with her nonreactive pupils, may have bled into her brain. This would also explain her comatose state and odd breathing pattern. Or she may have died from the gangrene affecting her arm. Without any way to obtain an autopsy, one never knows for sure.

On the other hand, not all snakebite victims die. Carlos, one of the Yaguas from across the stream, was cutting sugarcane one day when his hand came too close to an irritable fer-de-lance. His family called me to the worksite, which is coincidentally the same cane field in which the clinic now stands. I arrived within only forty-five minutes of the bite, but his hand was already nearly the size of a football (a North American, not a South American, football); I found not one, but two, sets of puncture marks on the bitten finger. With immediate antivenin—one vial—and antibiotics, however, he did well, except for a bit of bleeding around the gums and some bleeding in the soft tissues of his neck a few days later.

One fellow out on the Napo River tangled with a green tree-dwelling snake known locally as a *lorramachaco*, yet another member of the *Bothrops* genus. I happened to be out at Explorama's Napo Camp, fifty miles away from Yanamono, when the accident occurred. When I first saw him, he was feverish, dry and hot. His right middle finger was swollen and ugly, with a little slash at the darkened tip where someone had tried to extract the venom. Judging from the size of the finger (more or less like a bratwurst), and its color (dark purple), the extraction had not accomplished much. Thankfully, the erythema (redness) and edema (swelling) did not go much beyond the finger itself, though he said the severe pain extended up as far as his armpit. No one in the household possessed a watch or clock, but their best guess was that the bite had occurred a little over four hours earlier.

I broke out the antivenin and gave it. I cleansed the wound as well as I could under the circumstances, listened to his heart and lungs with a stethoscope to assure myself that he was not having an anaphylactic reaction to the antivenin, left antibiotics and instructions, and headed home.

On my follow-up visit the next morning, the man looked much more comfortable, although the fingertip remained discolored. At its tip, some purulent material of a rather attractive bright green shade had gathered. But this patient, too, healed well, and lived to tell the tale. So the doctors in the U.S., who have as much antivenin as they want, at any time of day or night, can debate the pros and cons of when and how to treat snakebite. I will continue to give antivenin even if the snakebite occurred more than twenty-four hours prior to my seeing the victim. But I will also continue to hope that such patients come to the clinic without delay, instead of pushing the limits of the antivenin's power.

And I will continue to be stingy with my limited stock—one or two vials per customer, please—unless I can find some other evidence that a lot more would be a lot better. And in that case, I will have to figure out how to get a lot more.

CHAPTER TWENTY

# Failures and Reflections

All of life involves a certain element of luck. You can be an honest, virtuous, industrious, careful person and still get hit by a drunken driver, or maybe worse, your husband or wife can be the victim. If it's not a drunken driver, then maybe it's a falling piano, or leukemia, or a problem child. But in the field of medicine, patients depend on more than their own luck. In the field of medicine, luck spills over from the doctor to the patient. Even the best surgeons encounter horrible cases in which anatomical irregularities or technical malfunctions or elementary errors, at any level of care, impede them and harm their patients. Even the best, the most intuitive and most compassionate pill-pushers occasionally run afoul of bacteria resistant to antibiotics, or unfavorable confounding circumstances. We are human and we err, especially when we are tired or distracted or sick ourselves. And it goes without saying that if the doctor is unlucky, his patient is doubly so.

I cannot claim to be one of the best. I know many doctors who are smarter than I. But I and my patients do seem, generally, to be lucky.

Life being what it is, however, there are exceptions.

One afternoon a man carried his eleven-year-old daughter into the clinic. The child had been ill for only two hours, with vomiting and diarrhea. He assured me that, prior to this crisis, she had been perfectly healthy. The family was worried not only about the suddenness of the illness, but perhaps even more disturbing, about the fact that she looked dreadful. She was barely conscious, with beads of sweat on her pretty face. An exam revealed nothing to localize the illness—no ear infection, no pneumonia, no rash, no stiff neck. Nothing. But she was very obviously very sick. There wasn't much to do, especially with no laboratory to help me make a clear diagnosis. I gave antibiotics and explained how to make oral rehydration fluid. I reassured the parents that it did not appear to be the cholera that they feared, and off they went.

At nightfall they returned. She had regurgitated everything they gave her to drink. Since severe dehydration can cause vomiting, which in turn leads to worse dehydration, administering intravenous fluid is usually an effective way of breaking the cycle. There was little else I could do, so I went with them to the house where they were visiting. The girl looked only slightly worse. I gave her a liter of intravenous fluid, and told her parents to work hard on getting more liquid into her orally. The next morning, an emissary came to tell me she had died during the night. The illness had lasted barely twelve hours. Worse, she died on her mother's birthday. Worse yet, her younger brother awoke at 6:00 A.M. with the same symptoms as his sister and died before noon. We were all disturbed by the suddenness of this mysterious illness. It was terrifying to the family to lose someone so young, with so little warning, and then her brother as well. (For all I know, more family members may have been affected later. The family lived elsewhere and were just visiting the area. They immediately fled home to bury their dead children. So I don't know whether or not more succumbed.)

I was also worried as a doctor, since I had absolutely no idea how to treat the patients or prevent other deaths. It appeared to be a contagious disease. What if it raced through the entire village? The only thing I could think it might be was meningococcus, a bacterium that can carry its victims off very rapidly. It hadn't really looked like meningococcus, but how could I know for sure? I didn't have enough penicillin or rifampicin to treat the entire neighborhood, but I did quickly give penicillin to the children in the house where the family had been staying, just in case. Then again, it might equally well have been typhoid, or some yet-unnamed jungle virus. No one will ever know.

Of course, even when the patient or doctor has lousy luck, the patient doesn't necessarily die. Sometimes he just suffers. I always tell my patients, who sometimes seem disappointed when they are told that they have nothing to worry about, that they do not want to be interesting cases. When it comes to medicine, it is much better to be normal, so dull that your physician must suppress a yawn. We doctors thrive on what we term "interesting cases." They are the spice in our lives, the source of exciting tales among us, but they are generally less fun, and sometimes nightmarish, for the patients involved.

One such "interesting case" began with a 3:15 A.M. knock on my door. A young man, imbibing heavily, had fallen off his stool onto a bottle and had sustained a bad cut on his back. The inch-deep laceration was three or four inches long, extending in a shallow V just below his left ribs. Something smooth was bulging out that might have been kidney. The victim was so inebriated that he could barely move, let alone cooperate. There was no air bubbling from the wound, and as well as I could tell, no significant collapse of the lung. I could have confirmed this fact more easily with him in a sitting position, but he could not sit up and there was no one around to help support him. His father had carried him here, but had soon after vanished into the night with a few other male relatives to resume their work of fishing. I was left alone with my patient, his girlfriend, who seemed about to faint, and his youthful sister-in-law.

I poked around in the depths of the gash but found nothing else. The alarmingly smooth bulge turned out to be only muscle. Even though I probed as deeply as I could, I encountered no broken ribs, and no entry into either the chest (lung) or the retroperitoneal space (where the kidney is located). I thought I had been able to penetrate the deepest extent of the cut, so I sewed him shut. It took a while.

He was still barely conscious by daylight. Once he woke up, he was going to have a hellatious hangover. His family carried him home, along with antibiotics and strict instructions to take him to the hospital in Iquitos immediately if he developed a fever, passed blood in his urine, or got worse in any way whatsoever.

He reportedly developed a fever a couple of nights later. I sent antibiotics, but other than that, could only repeat my instructions to get the lad into the city if he wasn't much, much better by morning. He wasn't. The next morning, the boy's grandmother came to the clinic, reporting that now he had pain in the lower left side of his chest. She requested a letter to take to the doctors in Iquitos. I would have preferred to examine him first, but she shook her head. He had too much pain to be moved any more than absolutely necessary. I hastily composed an outline of what had occurred, what I had done about it, and what medicines the young man was taking. Off she went, and I was left to ponder, had he ruptured his spleen? his kidney? As it turned out, neither was damaged.

I followed up on the young man and his family a few days later when I was in the city myself. He was at the older of the two city hospitals, which at night is easily mistaken for a POW camp. I passed down dim corridors and through deserted courtyards, and eventually found the young man in the surgery ward, lying pale on a sheetless mattress. His brother told me that he had received blood transfusions, which are a rarity here, so I surmised that his family must have been the donors. Further, his lung had been drained. I went to the nurses' station, hoping for a glimpse of his x-ray and his chart. The nurse gave me permission to look at his records when I explained that I was his original physician. The hitch was that the x-ray was not at the nurses' station, and the radiology department, where the film was stored, was closed at night. Period. The chart held a typical surgical note, as illegible as it was brief. I perused it carefully a couple of times, and discerned the diagnosis: hemothorax. The patient had a massive collection of blood leaking into the space between the lung and the chest wall. The chart did not say why this was occurring. No mention was made of a fractured rib, which would have explained it. I wished I could have gotten a peek at that x-ray, but it was out of the question.

I later heard from his relatives that the Iquitos doctors had drained the blood out of his chest. It filled up again. They drained it a second time; it accumulated yet again. At this point he had been running a high fever for a week. He was also septic, meaning that the infection had entered the bloodstream. This is a highly dangerous condition, sometimes fatal even today with potent antibiotics to combat such infections. Judiciously,  they operated and pulled out a chunk of bottle about an inch and a half long that had embedded itself deep in his lung, past the ribs and more than a few inches away from the entry wound. The piece of broken glass was buried in a welter of clotted blood, dying lung tissue and jaggedly slashed airways. Well, that certainly explained everything. He did heal well and recovered completely, although his family was faced with a medical bill that ran to a couple of hundred dollars, a huge sum around here.

Both of these cases—and there have been other failures, too—left me feeling inadequate. Doctors are human, and we sometimes err. I can accept that. But could I have done something else to save the girl and her brother from dying, or the young man from suffering for two weeks before finally receiving the necessary surgery? I am haunted by that thought. In those awful times when my patient dies despite my best efforts, I want very much to know why. Why? What is it that has killed them? Learning from my errors is seldom possible here, because there is no way for me to check my diagnosis.

It would have been great if on my initial exam I had discovered the glass buried in the young man's back, but realistically, that would have been tricky to say the least. The tissues had closed around the path of entry, and glass shards do not show up on an x-ray, even if I had one to look at. I realize that I might have missed the injury even at home in Wisconsin.

These two cases, however, illustrate some of the frustrations unique to my medical practice in the jungle. I have the training and the skill to do procedures that I simply can't risk in the jungle. For instance, I probably wouldn't have dared to drain the blood out of the young man's chest even if I had had the opportunity to properly examine him and discover the problem. Tapping the chest (draining fluid or air out) is a procedure that I have performed multiple times back in the U.S. But I wouldn't attempt it without a chest x-ray to assure me afterwards that I had not punctured the lung in the process, without a reliable source of suction to which to hook a chest tube if I did encounter a complication, and without blood available for a transfusion if needed. Sometimes I lack the elementary tools here to even make confident diagnoses. All the diagnostic aids available to modern physicians, such as blood studies, wound cultures, x-rays, ultrasounds, and electrocardiograms, are notably absent here.

Even more frustrating, perhaps, is not being able to attend to a hospitalized patient myself. In the U.S. the young man would have been "my" patient. That is to say, he would have been under my care, safely stashed in a hospital bed for me to monitor his x-rays, his urinalysis, and his fever. I would have had access to the laboratory and x-ray studies that tell me what is going on, and I would have had physical access to him. I would have been the one to find the hemothorax; I would have drained it; I would have begun to wonder what was really going on when it recurred; and when he developed a fever, I would have known about it and consulted with a surgeon. In this case, since I had not seen the young man since the night of his mishap, I was limited to sending his grandmother off with a preliminary letter on his condition.

It is frustrating when all I can do, in the most interesting cases, is to pass the patient on to some other doc with whom I cannot even communicate. It is terrible to feel useless and powerless.

When I send my patients to the city for treatment, I cannot even be sure that they will go there, because many are too poor to make the journey. I am also never absolutely certain that the physicians who will treat them are competent, that they will write any sort of report for me, or that my patients will deliver it to me if they do.

I hate being forced to choose between standing around doing nothing or violating the first dictum of medicine—"Do no harm"—by attempting risky procedures. When I do take a risk and all ends well, as with the cesarean sections I have done to date, I feel triumphant and accomplished and bold and adventuresome. But when all does not end well, I sometimes wish for the comfort of the shared responsibility that exists back in the Wisconsin medical world that I left.

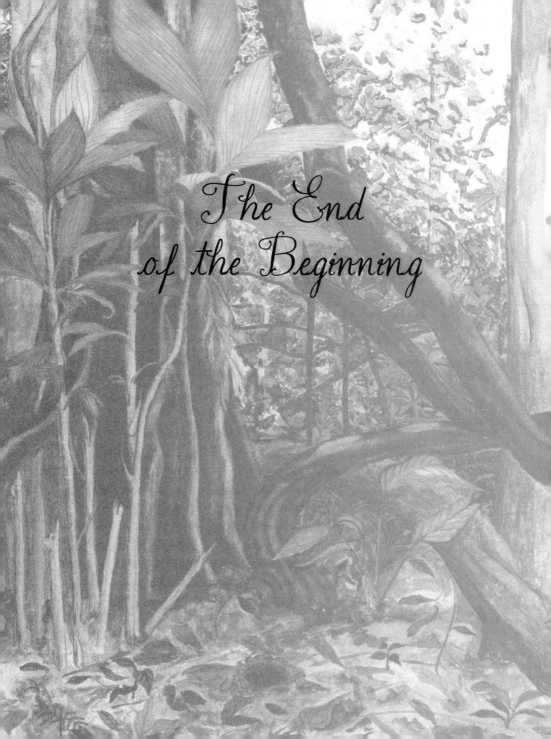

The End
of the Beginning

CHAPTER TWENTY-ONE

# Coming of Age

It took seven long years, but finally, after much striving, I am a real doctor—a real Peruvian doctor, that is. Here's how the miracle happened.

Coming as I do from the U.S. of A., where the legal climate is strict, it worried me from the very beginning that I had no actual license to practice medicine in Peru. I figured that my Wisconsin license would carry me for a while, since the state of legal affairs is more fluid here than in the U.S. Besides, I was practicing in an area where I was unlikely to come under official scrutiny, because no officials were to be found within many miles in any direction.

Nonetheless, in 1990 I began the process of seeking professional standing in Peru. I found that all I needed to do was to join the Colegio Médico del Perú—the Medical College of Peru (or CMP)—and receive a CMP number, which one proudly affixes to one's signature and all stamps and seals. The CMP is not a medical school as its name suggests, but the organization charged with documenting the legitimacy of physicians in this country. It is analogous to the bar for the legal profession; in Peru, CMP membership constitutes recognition that one has indeed trained as a physician. Easy, no?

The first hitch I encountered on my initial trip to the CMP in Iquitos was that it was closed for the month. I settled for requesting written permission from the local medical authorities, whose attitude was, "If you want to work in a place where we can't get our own doctors to go, and where there is so much need, thank you and more power to you." This would suffice for the time being.

A year or so later I was able to learn that I would have to present my case to the College's main office in Lima—a terrible idea from my perspective. Lima means an expensive plane flight and is a time-consuming jaunt from Iquitos. Instead, I wrote several letters to the CMP, hoping to take care of this via the mail. Not one of the letters yielded so much as acknowledgment that it had ever been received, let alone any more substantial response.

Finally, in mid-1993, I bit the bullet, bought a ticket, and boarded the plane. However, my trip only engendered more obstacles. To join the CMP, I would need a genuine, that is, Peruvian, medical degree. The one from the University of Wisconsin would count for nothing until it had been "revalidated," a task that could be performed only by the National Assembly of Rectors, whoever they were.

I wandered around the city until I finally located the headquarters of the rectors, only to be informed there that because the U.S. does not automatically recognize the validity of Peruvian medical degrees, Peru would not do so for U.S. degrees. They did offer me the information that I could try to get approval from the Ministry of Exterior Relations. A very kind woman in that office miraculously knew what I needed to do: go to the University of San Marcos in Lima (the oldest continuously functioning university in the hemisphere) and have them issue an approval. Thus, I made the first of what were to be many trips to downtown Lima. The friendly folks at San Marcos informed me that, fortunately for me, a set of rules had recently been promulgated to cover cases such as mine. In addition to paying a fee, I would be required to submit a formal request, my original University of Wisconsin medical degree, various and sundry stamped and notarized copies of my passport and my degree, and a transcript from the University of Wisconsin. To top it all off, they wanted a complete syllabus for every course I had taken in medical school. I retreated to the jungle and wrote to my friends in Wisconsin for help. By the time two of these friends, Dan and Judy Peterson, came to spend Christmas here in 1993, a suitably impressive list of syllabi had been dredged up, along with my full transcript, a copy of the dean's letter that goes out with every departing medical student, and all the other papers they could think of that looked impressive or that showed the university's seal. The weighty sheaf was about four inches thick. I could only hope that Spanish translations would not be demanded for every word of these documents, which were of course written in English. (Eventually translations were, in fact, required, and this cost a considerable sum of both money and time. In this case, however, only the money was mine, not the time.)

On January 4, 1994, I returned to Lima lugging a heavy briefcase. At this point a minor miracle occurred. While the Vatican will likely never officially recognize it as such, anyone who has spent any time dealing with Peruvian bureaucrats will recognize the event for what it was: the treasurer's office at Edificio Kennedy agreed over the phone to stay open past their regular working hours, in order to allow me time to arrive there and do my business. I was astonished, but thrilled. Otherwise, I would have had to spend the weekend in Lima, awaiting the arrival of Monday morning office hours. But they did in fact remain open and did meet with me, and the dean's office then advised me that I would hear from them shortly.

I went back to the clinic and settled down to wait. In late June, Explorama received a phone call from a Lima physician who had recently visited the lodge. He had interested himself in my case and had promised to check into it. "Come at once to Lima, your papers are approved," ran the message. So I hastened to Iquitos, packed bag in hand. Having lived in Peru now for four years, however, I cautiously made a phone call myself before purchasing my plane ticket, and sure enough, all was not quite in readiness. The first level of approval had indeed been achieved, but the all-important final signature was still lacking. I went back to my clinic and kept on waiting.

Toward the end of August, a fax showed up. Evidently the dean had authorized the revalidation of the title of Doctor of Medicine and Surgery for Doña Linnea Jean Smith, and requested that the rectors do the same. However, at just that moment a political scandal put the Assembly of Rectors in an uproar. None of them was signing anything for the time being. More months passed, as I waited somewhat less patiently. By now it was early 1995, a full year after I had handed over my heaps of paper to Dr. Piscoya, who had assured me that the entire process should take no more than three or four months. A kindly lawyer in Iquitos, whose firm also had an office in Lima, generously offered to carry on the quest, and took over the task of phoning Lima every week or two for the next year and a half. The committee in charge of "revalidations," however, just never could seem to get around to deciding to sign the already-approved papers.

Finally, in May of 1996, the lawyer flew to Lima to retrieve my original U.S. medical degree, languishing there all these months, and to retire my papers from the procrastinating office. On his arrival, the secretary reluctantly and sadly admitted to him that in fact all the papers (excluding, thank heaven, my degree, which was ensconced in her safe) had been lost, way back when the rectors were infighting and the new committee was being formed. Somewhere during the moving of offices, the box containing my papers had vanished. Yet, in all the phone calls passing back and forth during the preceding months, no one ever mentioned that simple fact. The apologetic secretary returned my degree, and promised to reconstruct my file with her own hands. After months in which she dug through old archives in search of copies of the missing documents, however, I finally heard that I no longer needed to go through the University of San Marcos. The

Universidad Peruana Cayetano Heredia, a private university in Lima with a well-respected medical school, had been authorized to grant approval to holders of foreign titles. I immediately switched strategies. In January 1997, six years after the start of this mission, I flew yet again to Lima and made my way to the Universidad Peruana Cayetano Heredia, where I was directed to a small window with an opening like a ticket booth. I explained my mission, and from behind the glass, a secretary slid a sheet of paper toward me which listed the requirements for revalidation of foreign medical degrees through the university. "Wait a minute," I said, "not so fast. As it happens, I have all these papers with me." (They were few enough, just the degree and a few supporting documents—no call for syllabi, or even transcripts, although I had armed myself with the latter, at least.) She then grudgingly gave me permission to enter the building, whereupon I approached her office from the interior. I handed everything over, was sent to the cashier's office to fork out the equivalent of about $800, and eventually spoke with a sympathetic woman who appeared to be the academic secretary and who promised that if my papers were indeed in order, the process should take no longer than six months (I had reported my previous experience in the matter, and her wry smile suggested she had heard it all before).

I again returned home and waited. But this time, not for long. A fax arrived in Explorama's office three scant weeks later, assigning a date for a meeting with the "Qualifying Judge," and in the first few days of February I flew again to Lima. My panel of judges were three distinguished-looking physicians, all male, and their interview was mainly one of congratulations interspersed with a few cursory medical questions. They were effusive in their praise for me and my work and were, they said, delighted that such a distinguished physician would come voluntarily to dedicate herself to their country. They assured me that the final stamps and seals would be speedily applied and that my revalidated degree would be forthcoming.

In fact, it was less than a month later that I received notice that a package had arrived for me. I hurried over from the clinic and opened it hastily. Inside was a copy of my degree—MY degree, in my name, with my photo on it—from the Universidad Peruana Cayetano Heredia. They did not merely approve my degree from the University of Wisconsin-Madison, they granted me one of their own. Not just an "honorary" type, either, but a genuine degree like they give to their own graduates, proclaiming that "having satisfactorily concluded her studies in the School of Medicine, Linnea J. Smith is hereby awarded the Degree of Physician-Surgeon." Thus, the University of Cayetano Heredia Medical School had done in two months what the other university could not bring itself to achieve in over four years. Now all I had to do was get registered with the CMP and I would be legal.

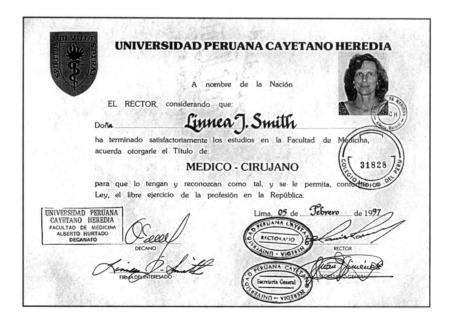

By this point, the actual *colegiatura*, or membership in the CMP, was somewhat anticlimactic. I merely needed to submit my newly acquired medical degree, my Wisconsin medical degree, a stack of forms, a bunch of signatures, another fee, a few more photographs, and a statement from the Department of Justice that I was not a wanted criminal (yes, truly), and the requisite processing was quickly performed. In June 1997 at the CMP in Iquitos, in the presence of several local medical dignitaries and the president of the Iquitos branch of the Colegio Médico del Perú, a small ceremony was held, with me as guest of honor. The dignitaries were seated behind a conference table that had been covered with a white lace cloth for the occasion. During the solemn, thankfully not too lengthy, ceremony, I was given a copy of the Physicians' Code to read aloud to the assembly. Several officers of the CMP gave short speeches. I solemnly pledged to uphold my duty and be a good doctor. Pam officially presented me with my new degree from Universidad Peruana Cayetano Heredia. The president then handed me the formal membership certificate with the CMP seal in gold, printing in red and blue, and my name in elegant calligraphy—"Linnea Jean Smith Richards"—with surnames from both of my parents, as is customary in all Hispanic countries. I was now legally entitled to sign myself Linnea J. Smith, C.M.P. 31828.

At last.

El

# Colegio Médico del Perú

**Por cuanto**, el médico cirujano

## Linnea Jean Smith Richards

ha cumplido con las disposiciones estatutarias y reglamentarias vigentes y está inscrito en el Registro Nacional de Matrículas, con el No. 31828

## Por tanto,

le expide el presente **Certificado**, que lo acredita como colegiado y lo faculta para el ejercicio de la profesión en el territorio de la República.

Lima, 31 de Mayo de 1997

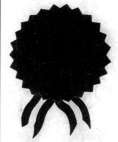

| | |
|---|---|
| DECANO | Dr. Francisco Sánchez Moreno Ramos |
| SECRETARIO DEL INTERIOR CONSEJO NACIONAL | Dr. Edgard Velarde Ponce |
| PRESIDENTE DEL CONSEJO REGIONAL | Dr. Mauricio Setomayor Menendez |
| SECRETARIO DEL CONSEJO REGIONAL | Dr. José Vera García |
| MEDICO CIRUJANO | Linnea J. Smith |

And how is the clinic doing these days?

The Clinic Yanamono is now, as of April 23, 1997, a United States registered nonprofit 501(c)(3) corporation and is free to accept tax-deductible contributions under the name Amazon Medical Project. For several years, St. John's Evangelical Lutheran Church in Prairie du Sac, Wisconsin, accepted donations on the clinic's behalf. But hundreds of people, many of whom have visited at Explorama and some who have not, asked repeatedly how they could support the ongoing operations of the clinic. Now the mechanism for receiving financial support is in place. This means that for the first time since 1990, I am earning a salary. I had never taken any personal expenses from the donations made to the clinic, because that didn't seem appropriate. But I cannot live forever on the savings left over from my Wisconsin working days, even with Explorama feeding me. So the board voted me a salary (now set at $600 a month), which makes me feel wealthy. A third of that will go to a retirement account so I will have, for the first time, a financial retirement plan. This is, of course, in addition to my primary retirement plan, which is that when the time arrives that I no longer feel like I can keep working, I will be bitten by a poisonous snake while walking in the forest. I still like my primary plan best, but it is nice to know that I won't have to depend on charity should I be unable to find a cooperative snake. The clinic is growing each year in its ability to serve the people of this region. Here are some data and comments from my 1997 Annual Report:

We saw a total of 2,436 patients this year. Of these, 2,078 received some kind of exam or other service (such as dental extraction), and the other 358 simply collected medicines. Among those who merely received medicines, some were picking up over-the-counter items like cough medicine, others were receiving treatment for their already diagnosed maladies such as malaria or leprosy, and some medicines were sent blindly to patients who really should have come in for examination but for one reason or another had not, and who might have died before they could do so, had I refused their family's plea for a hopefully suitable antibiotic to take home. That is not how it is done in the U.S., but at times there is not much choice here. We continue to see about 60 percent women versus 40 percent men, which is not surprising, and about two-thirds of our patients every year are adults, only one-third children, and that does surprise me, since children comprise over half of Peru's population. Family planning continues to be a big draw, however, so we are working on improving the ratio of children to adults.

We delivered our usual half-dozen babies this year, with no c-sections among them, much to my relief. There were forty-three cases of trauma, mostly minor but some, like burns, fairly grim.

We saw seventeen poisonous snakebites, with two fatalities among them, and the usual pneumonias and diarrheas (both major killers of small children) and skin problems, and did a dozen biopsies, generously analyzed by my friends back in Duluth. Malaria, virtually nonexistent when I first came here in 1990, continued the rise of the two previous years, this year producing ninety-three cases among our patients.

On the financial side, the clinic spent $28,762.33 in Peru, plus roughly $10,000 in salary and taxes and medical insurance and professional expenses for me. Employee salaries here in Peru accounted for about $18,000, including salary, benefits, one good meal a day, and taxes, for Juvencio, Edemita, and the three *huatchimanes*. We spent less than $3,000 on medicines, partly because of the generosity of the many visitors to Explorama who brought medicines with them for the clinic. (In fact, their generosity was such that I was able to forward quite a bit of medicine to the local government-run clinics, which are chronically short of supplies.) Income, of course, was mostly from the clinic's various U.S. supporters. The patients themselves provided only a little over $4,000 toward their own care. The balance was grass-roots support from family and friends, colleagues, tourists, organizations, foundations, and many generous individuals. Grants were provided by several Rotary chapters, Rotary International, and The International Foundation. Administrative services are donated by family and friends, so that all financial contributions can go directly to support delivery of medical services. Not shown on the balance sheet are the food and friendship provided to me free of charge by Explorama and its staff of employees, nor the love, moral support, and fruitcake from family and friends at home.

So what's new? Well, although I try to pretend that I never get tired, I do get to feeling worn out sometimes. This is due to several factors, the primary one being the wear and tear of always being on call. It's not that I work all the time; rather, it's the threat of being called to work for an emergency at any time. Because there is always—day or night, Sunday or holiday—the possibility of an emergency showing up on my doorstep, I can never quite relax completely. Of course, this is the way many country docs in the U.S. worked for years. Nevertheless, it can be fatiguing. With the help of my Iquitos accountant, however, we found a Peruvian physician willing to work for a few months, starting in early 1998. Another new development is the blood chemistry analysis machine purchased for the clinic by The International Foundation and on hold in Miami for months due to uncertainties about the customs end of things here. One goal this coming year is to get that equipment brought down here and set up in our clinic. Juvencio is taking on more responsibility, learning to do the clinic accounting and the simple statistical measures we try to maintain; he trades afternoons at the clinic with me, so that each of us gets a bit more time off and he gets a little more experience working solo. Management-wise I have a lot more responsibility now than in the old days, when leaving simply meant shutting the door and hanging out the "The Doctor Is Not In" sign. Of course I have a much more dedicated and skilled staff these days as well.

All this sometimes feels like a big responsibility for an icono-clastic renegade like me, running a clinic with no visible means of support. Fortunately, the invisible means are alive and well—thanks to all those whose donations have kept us going this far.

So that's the clinic's current status.

I am now a real Peruvian doctor, which means that my work here is finally legal and officially accepted.

The clinic is now an approved charitable foundation, which means that it can continue its work long after I'm gone.

And the clinic is busy and succeeding in its mission of caring for the medical needs of the wonderful people in this often overlooked and underserved region.

Had I dreamed it all up, I would never have dared to dream so much.

CHAPTER TWENTY-TWO

# What *Am* I Doing Here?

Eight years ago I left a comfortable group practice in rural Wisconsin and moved to a piece of Peruvian rainforest 2,300 miles up the Amazon River in order to develop an undersupplied, underfunded clinic. I am still here. Why?

When people ask me why I choose to live here, I think what they are really wondering is why a U.S.-trained physician, subject in the U.S. to unadulterated adulation and incalculable gross income, would leave all that in order to live sacrificially with minimal income and bury herself in this remote jungle without an evening newspaper, let alone the ten o'clock news or an occasional ice cream sundae.

It's a fair question, and I still don't have a very good answer. I'm always tempted to respond that I lost my U.S. medical license and I'm a fugitive from justice, or that I am a CIA spy assigned to protect U.S. interests, whatever they might be, in this remote corner of the world.

But the truth is that I like it here. This place, even after eight years, still seems magical to me. The people are warm and hospitable and handsome—beautiful women, winsome children, and chiseled men, with high cheekbones, ebony eyes, flashing smiles, and a love of dance. Although I will never exactly be one of them, being blonde and tall, an outsider by birth, and a medical doctor besides, they nonetheless invite me to their fiestas and raise no eyebrows when I am in their midst. They treat me with a mixture of friendship and respect that makes me feel loved. I don't claim not to suffer from the occasional bout of loneliness. But one can be lonely in Wisconsin, too, and I find it no more distressing to be lonely in this exotic location than in the place where I lived most of my life.

I guess I've always been a little eccentric. What many people might miss, I do not. When visiting in my native land, I occasionally go to a movie, or tour a museum, or even take in the theater. But I didn't do those things often when I was living in Wisconsin, and I do not miss them here. This is important. If I did value museums and newspapers and chocolate sauce, and left it all for the sake of the people I try to help here, then I would be, perhaps, a candidate for sainthood. But I don't much value those things. And although running the clinic is my work at the moment, I would never call myself noble. While it may be noble to suffer for a cause, it can hardly be called noble if it isn't suffering.

Don't I feel eternally like a stranger in a strange land? Far from it. This place is familiar. It felt like home the first week I arrived, and with time that feeling has only deepened. I have my house, my friends, and my work, which occupies most of my waking hours as well as some of my sleeping ones. I have the rain forest to walk in, and the city of Iquitos to visit for a change of pace.

In fact, I find it rather exciting to live here. As a child, I read voraciously. Now I, an alleged adult, get to live in one of the places just like the people in the novels I devoured years ago. Robert Louis Stevenson's characters have nothing on me. I have palms growing around my house, sometimes I see monkeys cavorting in them, and at certain times of the year, I go to and from everything—breakfast, lunch, dinner, work, visits to friends—in my genuine dugout canoe, carved by hand from a single log.

Like my favorite character, Huckleberry Finn, I get to go practically barefoot to work—no nylons or tight shoes for me (well, maybe Huck didn't exactly go to work, but he did generally run around shoeless). I work independently, for the most part, with no one except my own standards to tell me what to do . . . no quality control committees, here. Yes, it is sometimes maddening to be unable to help a patient for lack of simple materials, lack of basic diagnostic tools, lack of an expert to whom I can refer the patient for specialized help, lack of facilities, or lack of transport. Still, when I do manage to help, it feels all the more satisfying for having won against the odds.

But I must admit that my reasons go deeper. People often ask me what I miss most about home, and my response is always that I miss my family and my friends. I miss talking with my parents and seeing my nieces and nephews grow up. I miss medical conversations with my colleagues. I miss glorious afternoons in the Wisconsin hills on my bike.

But I don't miss television. I don't miss telephone tag. I don't miss volumes of news that is absolutely unaffected by my approval or disapproval of it. I don't miss traffic or shopping malls (though I'm grateful for conveniences like shampoo and decent flashlight batteries and cheap shoes, all of which I scarf up on forays into K-Mart when at home). I don't feel bad about not having a fancy car or a summer home. I don't care about matching dinnerware or living room sets. Those who know me from my pre-Peru days know how many of my possessions I've always either scrounged or made for myself, even when I was a real doctor and could afford to buy them. Furthermore, I'm not much bothered by some of the grittier realities of life here (such as peeing in the woods when visiting friends who have no bathroom).

I sometimes find the material wealth of my own country dismaying. I do not like being surrounded by so much stuff that I literally don't know what to do with it all. I am afraid that we North Americans are too often trapped by our wealth, partly because we have no conception of how much of it we have. We don't realize, for instance, that running water is a luxury—oh, sure, as luxuries go, it's pretty basic (and useful, and comforting, and healthful). But it is nonetheless a luxury, not a necessity. People lived without running water for thousands of years, and even today, less than half the world's population enjoys water piped into their houses—let alone multiple bathrooms or indoor and outdoor and upstairs and downstairs faucets.

How many of us would consider living in a home without a refrigerator, or without an oven? Yet, again, most—not just a sizable minority but a majority—of the world's human inhabitants do not have either—not to mention microwaves and telephones and Walkmans and personal computers and vacuum cleaners and lawn mowers.

But we do not—we cannot—see these things as luxuries. It is pretty much impossible when surrounded by all those appliances to recognize that not everyone lives as we and our neighbors do. I imagine the princes and princesses of the world grow up assuming that everyone lives in castles, complete with handmaidens and stables full of horses. I get tired of the addiction to things. It wears me down and makes me feel dissatisfied. I am appalled by the all-pervasive and ever slicker advertising that intrudes on every aspect of life in the U.S. Not that I am completely immune to this addiction to possessions. I get a kick out of a new pair of earrings or a new skirt; I enjoy tossing out something old and worn and replacing it with something fresh and new. I have wallowed for years in the pleasures of my clearly self-indulgent motorcycle. Still, by North American standards, I am shockingly unacquisitive.

Call it a genetic deficiency in "acquiring chromosomes." Again, this has nothing to do with sacrifice. I happen to like homemade bread, and homemade cookies, and homemade clothes, and homemade gifts. I find that manufactured items often disappoint me in their quality (with certain exceptions, such as the tools needed to make those homemade things), and they almost never meet my specifications. What use, for instance, is a skirt without pockets? and that looks just like what everyone else is wearing? I'd rather be different. I'd also rather make what I need myself, where possible, because I get a lot of fun out of the making or doing, I feel proud of myself when I finish, and I end up with enough money left over to run off and see the world—Peru, for instance.

Also, contemplating my own wealth and seeing that it is not universal makes me ethically uncomfortable. I don't seem to be able to forget the time when I was vacationing in the Virgin Islands, on a three-masted sailing ship (great fun, incidentally). We were served dinner on one of the islands, at a small, thatched-roof bar on the beach. There we were, piling our plates with fragrant roast pork and fresh fruits and black olives the size of plums—and in the shadows of the tropical night, outside the surrounding fence, skinny, desperate-looking children scuffled and peered through the palms and hoped for a leftover morsel or two. I am a glutton; I am selfish (if you don't believe me, ask my mother)—but I could not feel comfortable stuffing my own face with those hollow eyes staring at me. And whether I see them or not, those eyes are there, and I know it. I do not mean to be unappreciative of the country that reared me. I could not be here, playing Huckleberry Linnea, were it not for the education I received in the lush and beautiful state of Wisconsin. I probably could not be the independent cuss I am had I not been raised in a country where women do, at least most of the time, have opportunities that are by-and-large equal and in which a woman does not have to be regarded as chattel unless she wishes to be. I am grateful that I was raised by parents who share those values. I appreciate the shopping malls and hardware stores and the thousand sources of well-made, durable, high-quality material goods. Items ranging from rubber cement to good quality wrenches to underwear that doesn't fall apart at the first washing are difficult, even impossible, to obtain in Iquitos, let alone in the rain forest.

But when I am going home at sunset along the edge of the Amazon, listening to a toucan's ringing call floating out of the forest, I can't help but think that it sure beats traffic jams.

For all of these reasons, I am content here—at least for the moment.

What are my hopes and goals at this point? For the clinic, I wish the obvious: that it will continue after I am gone. Someday I will die, retire, or marry myself off, and when that day comes, I would like to leave knowing that what I have begun will endure.

This is, of course, easier said than done. I was delighted recently to finally find a Peruvian physician, just graduated from the small medical school in Iquitos, to work in the clinic for three months. Although temporary, he was a harbinger of the future: the first of what I hope will be a series of locally-trained medics who will strengthen the clinic's local base, receive for themselves a better opportunity for their early postgraduate training than they would likely have encountered in the underfunded, understocked, overworked government clinics, and form the nucleus of a web that will connect us to the Peruvian medical system. We also need a U.S. link. No matter how involved the clinic becomes with Peruvian physicians, nurses, and medical students, neither these people nor the clients of the clinic will ever be able to provide the funding needed to keep the clinic functioning. Thus we also need to develop an ongoing connection to the U.S., perhaps through a foundation for financial support and perhaps also through a series of U.S. docs, nurses, and students rotating through. Neither the foundation nor the rotating staff is yet in sight, but I keep hoping.

My personal goals are harder to identify. I do not imagine I will retire here. The city of Iquitos is too noisy, and without work, life here in the jungle would quickly become boring, not to mention difficult. There are no provisions made here for the infirmities of old age. Then again, at this point it is difficult to envision myself living permanently back in the U.S. So perhaps I will have to go with my original plan, and have that fatal encounter with a snake.

What can be concluded?

The challenge is exhilarating. It isn't always fun, and there are times when I question my judgment. But if you never take risks, you never know the satisfaction of success. And without either triumphs or losses, life would be very dull.

My life here is no great sacrifice in most of the ways significant to me. It still feels to me like an adventure. Mother Theresa I'm not, and I feel guilty when tourists exclaim something like, "How noble of you!" I simply have the good fortune to have a portable profession, a taste for the unusual, and a unique niche in which I can practice the one while indulging the other.

I just need to remind myself next time to be a little more careful about where I choose to go on vacation!

# Glossary of Spanish Terms

| | |
|---|---|
| aduana | customs office |
| aguardiente | strong liquor—lit. "burning water" |
| ambulante | walking street vendor |
| ampolla | ampule; an injection of medicine |
| auxiliare | nurse |
| bala | bullet |
| bijau | leaf used to wrap food |
| brujo | medicine man or shaman |
| buenas tardes | good afternoon |
| cajón | small box used as a percussion instrument |
| casa | house |
| cascavel | rattlesnake |
| chacra | field |
| chicha | alcoholic beverage made from cornmeal and sugar |
| clínica | clinic |
| coktel | beverage containing sugarcane rum, milk, beaten eggs, and vanilla |
| colegiatura | membership in the Colegio Médico del Perú |
| colectivo | river taxi |
| constancia | certificate |
| consulta | office visit |
| crisneja | thin, 8-foot pole used in roofing |
| cucaracha | cockroach |
| curandero | healer or herbalist |
| doctora | female doctor |
| empanadas | fried turnovers of *yuca* formed around chicken and vegetables |
| futbol | soccer |

| | |
|---|---|
| gringa/gringo | North American woman/man |
| huatchimán | watchman |
| juanis | balls of rice packed around seasoned chicken |
| Las Turistas | hotel in Iquitos, name meaning "the tourists" |
| madrina | godmother |
| maestra | teacher |
| maloka | communal house in a Yagua village |
| masato | alcoholic beverage made from *yuca* roots |
| miel | honey or sugarcane molasses |
| mijano | school of fish |
| motokar | motorcycle with back wheel replaced by small covered coach |
| motorista | driver |
| padrino | godfather |
| paiche | huge Amazon River fish prized as food |
| pamacari | thatched-roof boat |
| panetón | sweet bread sprinkled with dried fruit |
| pase | pass; Come in |
| pedido | request, petition |
| permiso | permission; May we enter? |
| Plaza de Armas | Military Square |
| pona | palm slat material used for flooring and walls |
| posta | rural medical center |
| pueblos jovenes | young towns |
| remedios | medicines |
| ribereños | river people; mestizos |
| sala | living room |
| sanitario | first-aid worker |

| | |
|---|---|
| señora | married woman |
| sin falta | without fail |
| solicitud | petition |
| tacacho | ball of mashed plantain, seasoned with salt and pork |
| tahuampa | swamp |
| tamales | ground corn and peanuts wrapped around meat, boiled in a leaf |
| tamshi | vines used in roofing |
| trago | drink; colloquially, strong liquor |
| trapiche | mill |
| velorio | vigil; wake |
| yuca | also known as cassava or manioc, a root crop that is a dietary source of starch |

## About the Author

Linnea Smith is a native of Wisconsin. At age 30, she entered the University of Wisconsin Medical School in Madison. After graduating and receiving board certification in Internal Medicine, she joined a small medical group in rural Wisconsin. She left that practice in 1990 to set up her remote jungle clinic on the banks of the Amazon River, three hours downriver from Iquitos, Peru.